RENAL DIET COOKBOOK

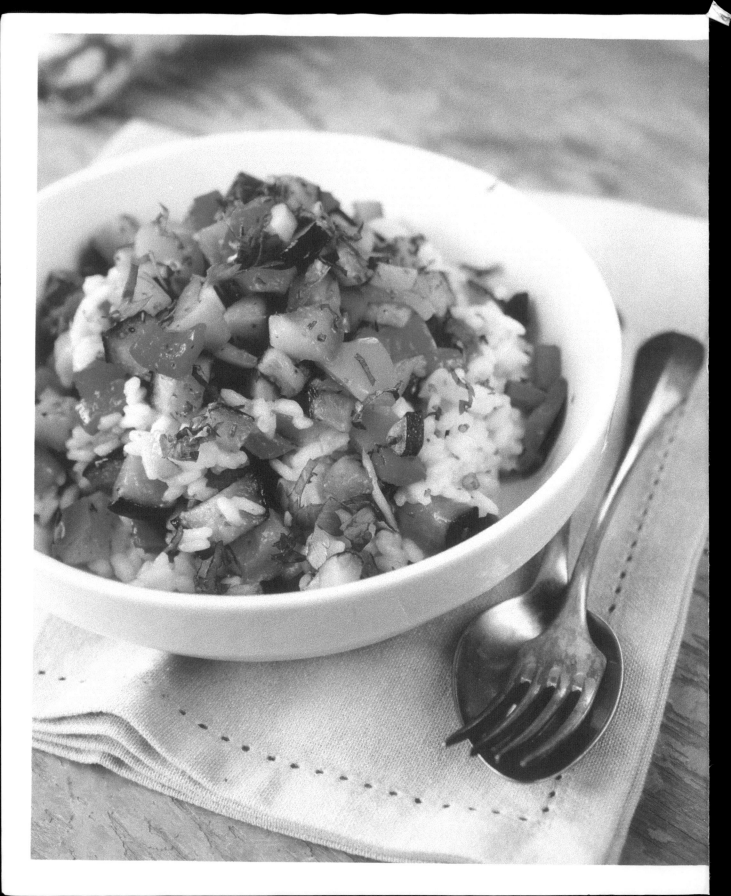

RENAL DIET COOKBOOK

THE LOW SODIUM, LOW POTASSIUM HEALTHY KIDNEY COOKBOOK

Susan Zogheib, MHS, RD, LDN

ROCKRIDGE PRESS

Front cover photo: Valerie Janssen/Stockfood. Back cover photos from left: Dave King/Stockfood; Davide Illini/Stocksy; Danny Lerner/Stockfood.

Interior photos: Mario Matassa/Stockfood, pg. 2; Keller & Keller Photography/Stockfood, pg. 6; Eising Studio–Food Photo & Video/Stockfood, pg. 8; Valerie Janssen/Stockfood, pg. 10; Renáta Dobránska/Stockfood, pg. 16; Kelly Knox/Stocksy, pg. 22; Tim Winter/Stockfood, pg. 40; Shutterstock.com, pg. 42; Melanie DeFazio/Stocksy, pg. 60; Gräfe & Unzer Verlag / Melanie Zanin/Stockfood, pg. 68; Katharine Pollak/Stockfood, pg. 82; Cameron Whitman/Stocksy, pg. 100; Food and Drink Photos / Simone Vogel/Stockfood, pg. 120; Dave King/Stockfood, pg. 138; Jo Kirchherr/Stockfood, pg. 152; Davide Illini/Stocksy, pg. 166; Valerie Janssen/Stockfood, pg. 186 Jonathan Gregson/Stockfood, pg. 202; Danny Lerner/Stockfood, pg. 220; Keller & Keller Photography/Stockfood, pg. 238.

ISBN: Print 978-1-62315-661-9 | eBook 978-1-62315-662-6

R1

5 DIET TIPS
FOR HEALTHIER KIDNEYS

By now, you have probably learned quite a bit about chronic kidney disease. You may have symptoms or you may not. The good news? There are many ways you can slow down its progression and take back some control. Here are five specific steps you can take to help you feel better and preserve your kidney function.

1. **Limit the amount of salt (sodium) in your diet.** Monitor your sodium intake and maintain a healthy blood pressure below 140/90 mm Hg. Eat more fresh vegetables and fruits, which are naturally low in sodium. Cut back on high-sodium foods, such as processed foods, fried foods, deli meats, and soy sauce. Aim for less than 2,300 milligrams of sodium each day.

2. **Lose excess weight, if needed.** Ask your physician or registered dietitian to determine your body mass index, also known as BMI. BMI is a measure of body mass based on height and weight that applies to adult men and women. If your doctor advises you to lose weight, make that a priority.

3. **Select foods with lower levels of phosphorus.** Low-phosphorus foods can help protect your bones and blood vessels. Nowadays, a lot of food products have added phosphorus. Check ingredient labels for phosphorus or words with "phos" in them.

4. **Eat the right amount of potassium.** This will help your nerves and muscles work the proper way. If the potassium level in your blood is high, avoid salt substitutes because they can be very high in potassium. Other foods rich in potassium include dark green leafy vegetables, tomatoes, potatoes, oranges, orange juice, bananas, dried fruit, and melons.

5. **Make heart-healthy food choices.** A diet filled with lean meats, chicken, turkey without the skin, fish, and whole grains in moderation will go a long way toward maintaining health. Meat, fish, and poultry portions should be kept to about 3 ounces, or the size of a bar of soap.

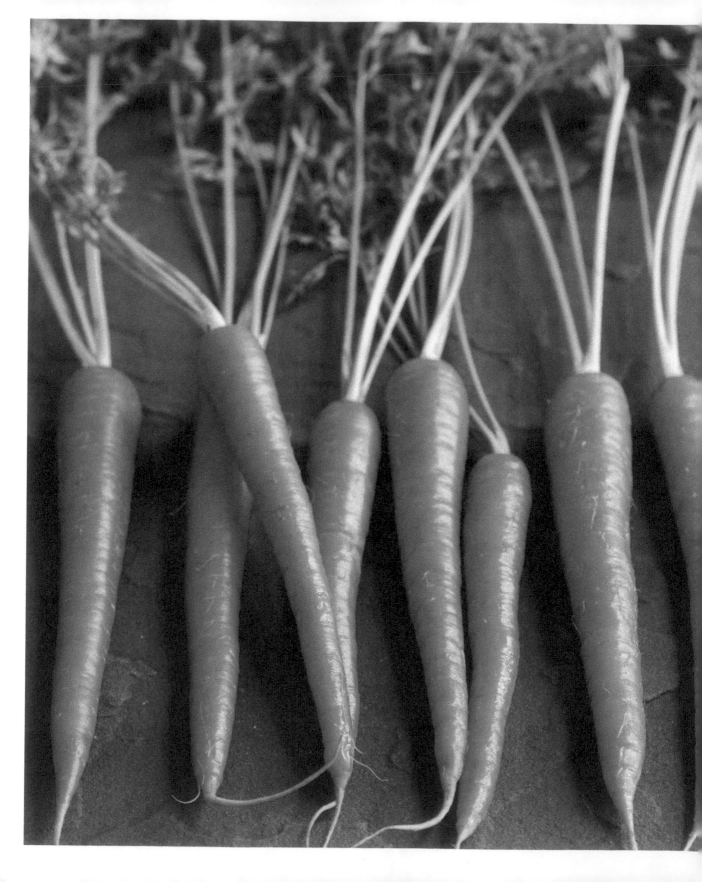

I dedicate this book to
all my patients at DaVita.
Sometimes I inspire you;
more often, you inspire me.

CONTENTS

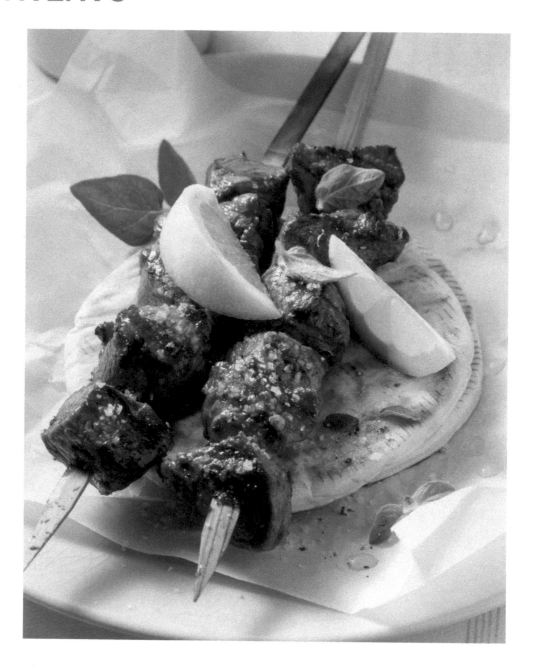

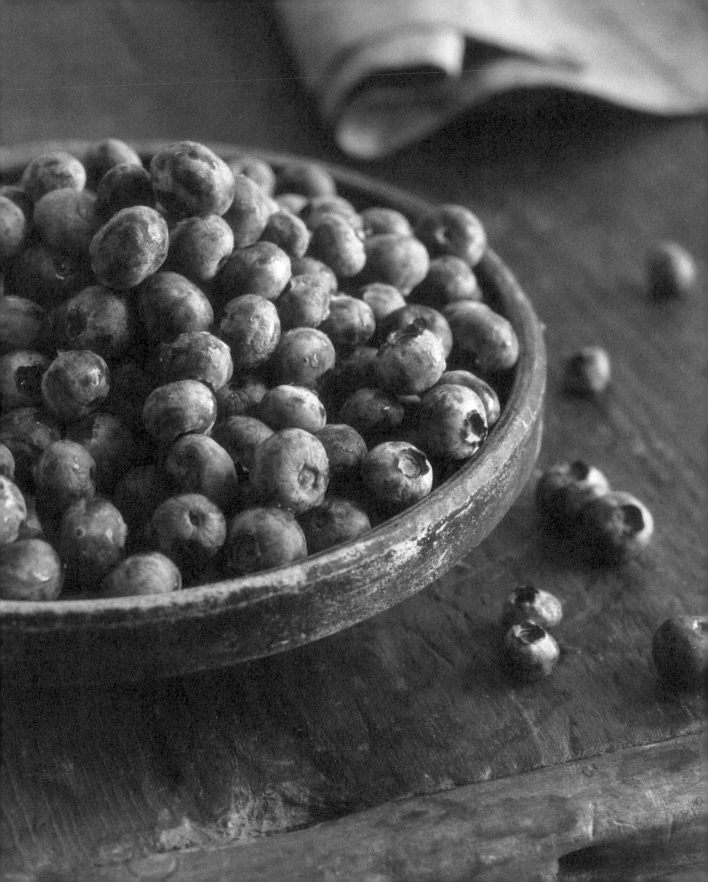

FOREWORD

The lifestyle choices we ask of our patients to maintain their health is vital. Among complex diseases, patients with kidney disease have specific needs—nutrition being one of the most important. As a nephrologist, I have told my own patients to "watch what you eat" knowing full well just how hard it is to cut back on the amount of salt in their diet, avoid foods that are high in potassium, or restrict their phosphorus and fluid intake. Those restrictions essentially take a lot of choice and "flavor" out of their lives.

This is what I love about Susan's approach in this book. A nutrition expert with over a decade of experience taking care of patients, she simply makes the diet easy and satisfying. As you read her book, it will probably surprise you that a renal diet can look and taste so good while still being healthy. While proper nutrition may not be something that your body responds to immediately, adhering to a renal diet is likely to greatly reduce the chances of having more kidney complications or being hospitalized. Susan has done a masterful job in educating patients about their disease, explaining why watching your diet is important, and offering meal plans and recipes that encourage compliance and fun—information that can make a huge difference in their lives.

John Wigneswaran, MD
Vice President Clinical Affairs
DaVita Healthcare Partners

INTRODUCTION

You're not alone. According to the National Kidney Foundation, 26 million American adults have chronic kidney disease. Millions of others are at high risk or have signs of the disease and don't know it.

Chronic kidney disease is not reversible, but you can learn what options are available to prevent it from getting worse. Your most effective method of prevention? Your diet.

As a renal dietitian, my job is to teach you how to take a proactive role in your health and eat better so you can continue to lead a productive and active life. The health of your kidneys is greatly affected by your diet, so it is important to know which foods are best to eat and which ones may cause problems. A proper renal diet controls the amount of protein, sodium, potassium, and phosphorus that you consume. Following this diet can help decrease the amount of waste made by your body, which can reduce your kidneys' workload and possibly preserve kidney function. The renal diet may help prevent the disease from progressing to the next stage and help delay total renal failure or dialysis by many years.

It can be quite overwhelming to think about what to eat on a low-protein, low-sodium, low-potassium, and low-phosphorus diet. It's not as simple as making one small change or eliminating a couple types of foods from your diet. This book takes the mystery and the stress out of figuring out recipes, as well as what to choose from the menu when you dine out. Most importantly, it will help you succeed at maintaining the dietary changes for the long term.

A restrictive renal diet can be both delicious and imaginative; you're not banished to years of bland foods. The 28-day meal plan in chapter three will help get you started. Some of the recipes even include modifications to accommodate individuals with end-stage renal disease or those who are receiving dialysis.

When it comes to a renal diet, it is important to arm yourself with knowledge. Consider me your personal dietitian and cheerleader in the days ahead. Stay positive and do your best to stick to the 28-day plan—and beyond—and you will be on your way to healthier, happier kidneys. You can do it!

Susan Zogheib, MHS, RD, LDN

PART

1

KIDNEY DISEASE AND DIET

CHAPTER ONE

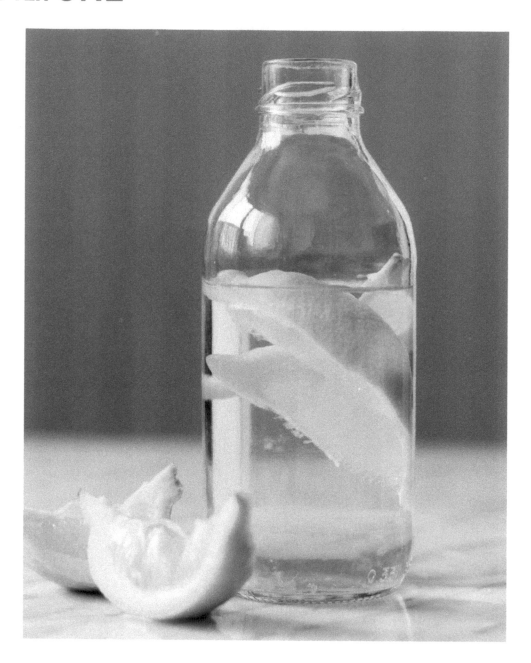

UNDERSTANDING KIDNEY DISEASE

When you educate yourself about chronic kidney disease, you will feel more empowered and less scared about living with the disease. You can take back control of your life! What you eat and the lifestyle choices you make are very important. If you are diagnosed in the early stages of the disease, there are many steps you can take to prolong your kidney function. When you make positive changes, have patience, and commit to working closely with your health-care team, chances are very good that you will be able to enjoy a high-quality, happy, and active life.

What Is Kidney Disease?

Let's begin by understanding how kidneys function. Your body has two kidneys that are bean-shaped and about the size of your fist. They can be found in the middle of your back, on the left and right of your spine, just below your rib cage. When the kidneys are working properly, they help keep your whole body in balance by doing the following very important jobs:

1. Clean waste materials from your blood

2. Remove extra water from your body

3. Regulate your blood pressure

4. Stimulate your bone marrow to make red blood cells

5. Control the amount of calcium and phosphorus absorbed and excreted

When you have chronic kidney disease, your kidneys do not work properly and cannot do these jobs. Although there is no cure for kidney failure, it is very possible to live a long and healthy life with proper treatment and good dietary and lifestyle choices.

Causes

Kidney disease is most often caused by poorly controlled diabetes or high blood pressure. Physical injury and drug toxicity can also damage your kidneys. Kidney disease affects people of all ages and races, but African Americans, Hispanics, and Native Americans tend to have a greater risk of kidney failure. This is mostly due to a higher incidence of diabetes and high blood pressure in these populations.

Uncontrolled diabetes is the leading cause of kidney failure. In fact, 44 percent of people who start dialysis have kidney failure caused by diabetes. Diabetes develops when blood glucose (blood sugar) levels are too high in the body. When our bodies digest protein from the food we eat, the process of digestion creates waste products. In the kidneys, millions of tiny blood vessels, called capillaries, act as filters. As blood flows through the capillaries, the waste products are filtered out into our urine. Substances such as protein and red blood cells are too big to pass through the capillaries and stay in the blood.

Diabetes damages this process. High levels of blood sugar make the kidneys filter too much blood. All the extra work wears down the filters, and after many years the filters start to leak. The good protein our bodies need is then filtered out and lost through the urine. Eventually, the kidneys cannot remove the extra waste from the blood. This ultimately leads to kidney damage or failure. This damage can happen over many years without any signs or symptoms. That is why it is so important for people with diabetes to manage their blood-sugar levels and get tested for kidney disease periodically.

High blood pressure is another contributor to kidney disease. One in three Americans with high blood pressure, also known as hypertension, is at risk for kidney disease. High blood pressure is the second leading cause of kidney disease, and increases your risk of developing a heart attack or stroke. Treatment and lifestyle changes, including blood-pressure medications, following a healthy diet, and exercising can lower blood pressure.

High blood pressure means the heart has to work harder at pumping blood. As time passes, high blood pressure can harm blood vessels in your body, including the ones in your kidneys—causing them to stop filtering out waste and extra fluid from your body. The extra fluid in your blood vessels can also make your blood pressure rise, creating a vicious and detrimental cycle. As in diabetes, this damage can happen over many years without any signs or symptoms. It is very important for people with high blood pressure to control their blood pressure and get tested for kidney disease, just like people who have diabetes. High blood pressure is the cause of more than 25,000 new cases of kidney failure in the United States every year.

Symptoms

Kidney failure is a progressive disease; it does not happen overnight. Some people in the early stages of kidney disease do not show any symptoms. Symptoms usually appear in the later stages of kidney disease. Some people may not even show any symptoms of kidney disease until their kidneys fail (end stage).

When the kidneys are damaged, wastes and toxins can build up in your body. Once the buildup starts to occur, you may feel sick and experience some of the following symptoms:

Nausea	Itching	Swelling of your feet and ankles
Poor appetite	Weight loss	
Weakness	Muscle cramps (especially in the legs)	Anemia (low red blood cell count)
Trouble sleeping		
Tiredness		

The good news is that once you begin treatment for kidney disease, your symptoms and general health will start to improve.

Five Stages of Chronic Kidney Disease

There are five stages of chronic kidney disease, each differentiated by the amount of kidney damage and glomerular filtration rate, a measure of how well the kidneys are working. Stage 1 is the least severe and comes the closest to healthy kidney function, while stage 5 requires dialysis or kidney transplant. Your physician will determine your treatment based on which stage of kidney disease you have. Talk to your doctor if you have any questions about your stage of kidney disease or treatment.

Five Stages of Chronic Kidney Disease

STAGE	DESCRIPTION	GLOMERULAR FILTRATION RATE (GFR)
Normal kidney function	Healthy kidneys	90 mL/min or more
Stage 1	Kidney damage with normal or high GFR	90 mL/min or more
Stage 2	Kidney damage with mild decrease in GFR	60–89 mL/min
Stage 3	Moderate decrease in GFR	30–59 mL/min
Stage 4	Severe decrease in GFR	15–29 mL/min
Stage 5	Kidney failure	Less than 15 mL/min or receiving dialysis

Frequently Asked Questions

Do high-protein diets cause kidney disease?

A high-protein diet may actually make kidney function worse in people who are in the early stages of kidney disease. However, for most people with healthy kidneys, a high-protein diet is not harmful, especially if followed for only a short period of time. The long-term consequences of following a high-protein and carbohydrate-restricted diet are still being studied.

Is soda bad for my kidneys?

Many dark sodas, except for most brands of root beer, should be avoided. They contain phosphorus additives, which are absorbed 100 percent by the body. Make sure to check food labels for ingredients containing phosphorus. Replace dark sodas with 7UP, Cherry 7UP, cream soda, ginger ale, Sprite, or acceptable root beers. Although these sodas contain less phosphorus, it is still a good idea to limit the amount of soda you drink to reduce the amount of empty calories; soda does not provide your body any nutritional value.

What kind of vegetables can I eat if my chronic kidney disease is stage 3?

If you have stage 3 chronic kidney disease, you have moderate kidney damage. Limiting some vegetables is important if blood tests show that your potassium levels are above normal. Some of the best options for vegetables to eat are the following: broccoli, cauliflower, celery, cucumbers, asparagus, eggplant, and raw spinach. Make sure to keep portion sizes to ½ cup with about two to three servings each day.

Is it possible to have low-sodium hot dogs or cold cuts once in a while for lunch or at a cookout?

Hot dogs and deli meats are high in phosphorus, so portion sizes play an important role in controlling your phosphorus intake. For example, if your phosphorus level is below goal or within goal consistently, incorporating hot dogs and deli meats a few times a month may be suitable for you.

Are there any kinds of cheeses that patients with kidney disease are able to eat?

Cheese contains large amounts of phosphorus. Some cheeses are lower in phosphorus than others, including cream cheese, natural cheddar, Swiss, and Brie. One to two ounces of cheese is usually the recommended amount in a low-phosphorus diet.

CHAPTER TWO

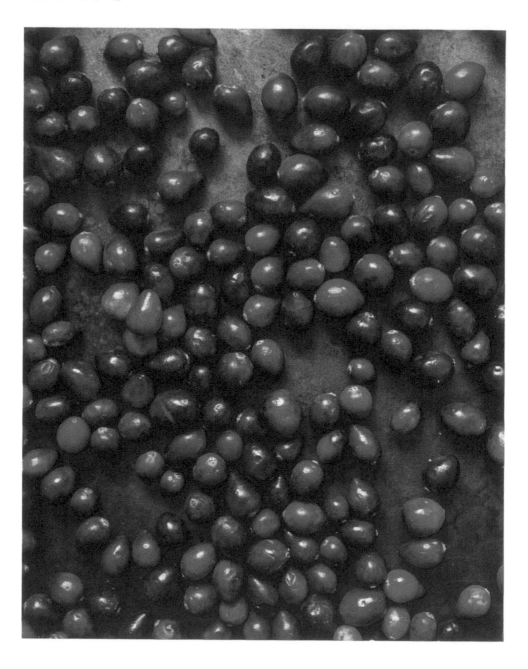

THE DIET CONNECTION

Y ou've made the commitment to eating better. Congratulations! Making healthy food choices is important to everyone, but it is especially important if you have chronic kidney disease. There are many benefits to making healthy food choices. Good nutrition gives you energy for daily living, prevents infection, builds muscle, helps you maintain a healthy weight, and may help your kidneys from getting worse. Good nutrition will help you avoid complications of renal disease, such as fluid overload, high blood phosphorus, high blood potassium, bone disease, and weight loss.

Key Diet Concerns

Depending on the stage of your kidney disease, type of treatment, blood-work results, and whether you have diabetes or high blood pressure, your renal diet "prescription" will vary. Following a renal diet may seem over-whelming at first, but it is easier to follow than you think. The 28-day diet plan outlined in this book will give you a great start and provide you with delicious, kidney-friendly recipes.

This chapter outlines the following very important macronutrients, vitamins, and minerals, which should be carefully monitored to keep your kidneys as healthy as possible:

Potassium	Protein	Carbohydrates
Phosphorus	Fats	Vitamins/Minerals
Calories	Sodium	Fluids

As you read this chapter, please keep in mind that *serving size* is the bottom line for whether a food is low, moderate, or high in a given nutrient. For example, if you eat a large bowl of raspberries instead of a half-cup serving, a low-potassium food has now become a high-potassium serving of that food.

Potassium

Potassium is an important mineral that is needed for the body to keep your heart strong and healthy. It is also needed to keep the water balance between your cells and body fluids in check. Healthy kidneys remove excess potassium through urination. When the kidneys are not functioning properly, they cannot remove the potassium, so it builds up in the blood.

Having too much or too little potassium in the blood can be harmful to the body. While some people with kidney disease need more potassium, others need less. Depending on how well your kidneys are functioning, your potassium need may vary.

All foods contain some potassium, but some foods contain large amounts of potassium. On the following pages is a table that lists low-potassium, medium-potassium, and high-potassium foods. If you have chronic kidney disease, the amount of potassium you eat is not usually restricted unless your blood potassium level is high. Please talk with your physician about having your blood potassium level checked. And if you are receiving dialysis, your potassium intake should be kept between 2,000 and 3,000 milligrams per day.

Potassium in Common Foods*

LOW POTASSIUM (Less than 150 mg/serving)	MEDIUM POTASSIUM (151–250 mg/serving)	HIGH POTASSIUM (More than 251 mg/serving)
Alfalfa seeds, sprouted, raw	Apple, without skin, 1 large	Apricot, 1 cup
Applesauce, sweetened	Apricots, in heavy syrup, drained	Artichoke, 1 medium
Apple juice	Apricot, halves, 1 medium	Avocado
Bagel, 1 plain (4-inch diameter)	Asparagus, 5 boiled spears	Bamboo shoots, cooked
Beans, green, frozen	Beans, green, boiled, 1 cup	Banana, 1 small
Blueberries	Blackberries, 1 cup	Beans, black, mature, boiled
Cabbage, shredded, boiled	Broccoli, frozen, 1 cup	Beans, Lima, large, mature, boiled, ⅓ cup
Carrot, baby raw, 1 medium	Brussels sprouts, boiled	Beans, pinto, mature, boiled
Cherries, sour canned, in syrup	Carrots, sliced, 1 cup	Beans, refried, canned
Coffee, 1 cup	Cereal, All-Bran	Beets, cooked
Cranberries, dried	Cherries, 10 sweet	Cabbage, Chinese, cooked
Cranberry juice	Chickpeas, dried, boiled	Cantaloupe, cubed, 1 cup
Cranberry sauce, canned	Collards, chopped, frozen	Chard, Swiss, boiled, ⅓ cup
Eggplant, boiled	Corn, yellow, boiled, 1 ear	Chocolate
Fig, raw, 1 medium	Date, dried, 1 date	Dates, medjool
Ginger ale, 12 ounces	Elderberries	Beans, dried
Grapes	Grape juice, 1 cup	Fruits, dried
Lemon, 1 medium	Grapefruit juice	Mango, pieces, 1 cup
Lime, 1 medium	Grapefruit, ½ medium	Milk, 1%, 1 cup
Mustard greens, frozen	Honeydew melon, pieces	Milk, soy 1 cup
Oatmeal, regular	Kiwifruit, 1 medium	Milk, whole, 1 cup
Okra, cooked	Leeks, 1 raw	Molasses, 1 tablespoon
		Mushrooms, cooked, 1 cup

▶

*One serving = ½ cup unless otherwise noted.

Potassium in Common Foods* *(continued)*

LOW POTASSIUM (Less than 150 mg/serving)	MEDIUM POTASSIUM (151–250 mg/serving)	HIGH POTASSIUM (More than 251 mg/serving)
Onions, raw, diced	Mustard greens, cooked, ¾ cup	Nectarine, 1 medium
Parsley, raw, 10 sprigs	Onion, chopped, boiled	Nuts, mixed, 2 ounces
Peaches, canned, in syrup, drained	Orange, 1 medium	Orange juice, fresh
Pears, canned, in syrup, drained	Peach, 1 small	Papaya, 1 small
Peppers, sweet, cooked	Pear, 1 medium	Plantain, sliced, cooked
Pineapple, pieces	Peppers, hot chili	Pomegranate, 1 small
Plum, 1 medium	Peppers, sweet, raw	Pomegranate juice
Popcorn, buttered	Pineapple juice	Potatoes, white, baked, 1 medium
Prunes, dried, 1 prune	Pineapple, canned	Raisins, seedless, 1.5-ounce box
Radicchio, raw, shredded	Prickly pear, 1 medium	Sapodilla, 1 medium
Raspberries	Prunes, canned, 5 prunes	Sauerkraut, undrained, 1 cup
Rhubarb, cooked with sugar	Radishes, raw, sliced, 1 cup	Spinach, cooked
Rice, white, enriched, 1 cup cooked	Raspberries, frozen, sweetened, 1 cup	Succotash, boiled
Spaghetti, enriched, cooked	Scallions, chopped, raw, 1 cup	Sweet potatoes, boiled
Spinach, raw, chopped	Squash, summer	Tomato, 1 medium
Tea, black, 8 ounces	Strawberries, whole, 1 cup	Tomato paste, canned, ¼ cup
Turnips, white, cubed	Tangerine, 1 large	Tomato sauce, canned, ¼ cup
Water chestnuts, canned	Tortillas, corn, 4 (6-inch diameter)	Water chestnuts, raw
Watermelon, pieces	Turnip greens, chopped	

*One serving = ½ cup unless otherwise noted.

Phosphorus

Phosphorus is a naturally occurring mineral. Phosphates are salt compounds containing phosphorus and other minerals, and these are found in our bones. Along with calcium, phosphorus helps build strong and healthy bones. Healthy kidneys are able to remove extra phosphorus in the blood. Virtually all foods have phosphorus or phosphate additives, so it is difficult to completely eliminate it from your diet.

Foods that naturally contain high levels of phosphorus include milk and dairy products, amaranth, bran, brown rice, millet, quinoa, dried beans and peas, nuts and seeds, organ meats, sardines, beer, and chocolate. Foods that have a lot of phosphate additives include some types of baking powder, pancakes, waffles, biscuits, baked goods, instant puddings and sauces, processed and enhanced meats, bottled iced teas, and sodas.

If you have too much phosphorus in your blood, calcium is pulled from your bones, resulting in weak bones. When the kidneys are failing, phosphorus builds up in the blood and may cause problems such as severe itching, muscle aches and pain, bone disease, and hardening of the blood vessels, including those leading to the heart, as well as deposits on the skin and in the joints.

The table on the following pages lists low-phosphorus, medium-phosphorus, and high-phosphorus foods. Please talk with your physician about getting your blood phosphorus level checked. For people with chronic kidney disease and those who are receiving dialysis, phosphorus in the diet should be limited to between 800 and 1,000 milligrams per day.

Phosphorus in Common Foods*

LOW PHOSPHORUS (Less than 150 mg/serving)	MEDIUM PHOSPHORUS (151–250 mg/serving)	HIGH PHOSPHORUS (More than 251 mg/serving)
Apple	Beans, black, 1 cup	Peanuts, oil roasted, 2 ounces
Bagel, 1 plain (4-inch diameter)	Beans, fava, 1 cup	Almonds, oil/dry roasted, 2 ounces
Barley, pearled, cooked	Beans, kidney, 1 cup	Baked beans, 1 cup
Beans, green	Beans, pinto, 1 cup	Beans, small white, mature, boiled, 1 cup
Bread, pita, 1 (6.5-inch diameter)	Beef, bottom round, 3 ounces	Beef, liver, cooked, 3 ounces
Bread, pumpernickel, 2 slices	Beef, chuck roast, 3 ounces	Beefalo, 3 ounces
Bread, white, 2 slices	Beef, eye round, 3 ounces	Buttermilk, 1 cup
Butter, 1 tablespoon	Beef, ground, 70% lean, 3 ounces	Calamari, fried, 3 ounces
Cabbage	Beef, ground, 95% lean, 3 ounces	Cashews, dry roasted, 2 ounces
Cauliflower	Beef, sirloin steak, 3 ounces	Cereal, bran, 100%
Cereal, crispy rice, 1 cup	Black-eyed peas, 1 cup	Cereal, wheat germ, ¼ cup
Cheese, Brie, 1 ounce	Bread, whole wheat, 2 slices	Cheese, goat, 2 ounces
Cheese, feta, 1 ounce	Catfish, breaded/fried, 3 ounces	Cheese, parmesan, 2 ounces
Cocoa, unsweetened, 2 tablespoons	Cheese, blue, 2 ounces	Cheese, ricotta, part skim
Cookies, shortbread, 4	Cheese, cheddar, 1 ounce	Cheese, Romano, 2 ounces
Cornflakes, 1 cup	Cheese, mozzarella, 1 ounce	Chia seeds, 1 ounce
Cottage cheese, nonfat	Cheese, provolone, 2 ounces	Chicken, liver, cooked, 3 ounces
Couscous, cooked	Cheese, Swiss, 1 ounce	Clam chowder, New England
Cream cheese, 1 ounce	Chicken, breast, 3 ounces	Clams, cooked with moist heat, 3 ounces
Cucumber		
Duck, with skin, 3 ounces		

*One serving = ½ cup unless otherwise noted.

Phosphorus in Common Foods*

LOW PHOSPHORUS (Less than 150 mg/serving)	MEDIUM PHOSPHORUS (151–250 mg/serving)	HIGH PHOSPHORUS (More than 251 mg/serving)
Egg white, 1 large	Chicken, dark meat, 3 ounces	Corn bread, 1 piece
Egg yolk, 1 large	Chickpeas, 1 cup	Crab, Alaska king, cooked with moist heat, 3 ounces
Eggplant	Chocolate, plain, 2 ounces	Custard, flan, 1 cup
English muffin, 1 plain	Cod, Pacific, 3 ounces	Flounder, 3 ounces
Figs	Cottage cheese, 1% fat	Halibut, Atlantic/Pacific, 3 ounces
Gelatin, water base	Cottage cheese, 2% fat	Lentils, mature, boiled, 1 cup
Ginger ale, 1 can	Crab, blue, cooked with moist heat, 3 ounces	Milk, 1%, 1 cup
Grapefruit	Crab, Dungeness, cooked with moist heat, 3 ounces	Milk, chocolate, 1 cup
Grapes	Lamb, kabobs, domestic, 3 ounces	Milk, evaporated, nonfat
Grouper	Lamb, leg roast, domestic, 3 ounces	Milk, nonfat, 1 cup
Hominy grits	Lamb, New Zealand, 3 ounces	Milk, whole, 1 cup
Ice cream, 10% fat, vanilla	Lobster, cooked with moist heat, 3 ounces	Mussels, blue, cooked with moist heat, 3 ounces
Lettuce	Macadamia nuts, 3 ounces	Nuts, brazil, 2 ounces
Milk, soy, 1 cup	Milk, canned, sweetened, condensed, ¼ cup	Nuts, pine, 2 ounces
Oatmeal, cooked, 1 packet	Mushrooms, cooked, 1 cup	Oysters, Eastern, cooked with moist heat, 3 ounces
Onions		Peanuts, boiled, 1 cup
Oysters, canned, 3 ounces		Peanuts, dry roasted, 3 ounces
Oysters, raw, Pacific, 3 ounces		Peanuts, oil roasted, 2 ounces
Pasta, 1 cup		
Peas, split, mature, boiled		
Plums		

*One serving = ½ cup unless otherwise noted.

▶

Phosphorus in Common Foods* *(continued)*

LOW PHOSPHORUS (Less than 150 mg/serving)	MEDIUM PHOSPHORUS (151–250 mg/serving)	HIGH PHOSPHORUS (More than 251 mg/serving)
Popcorn, air-popped, 1 cup	Mussels, raw, blue, 3 ounces	Pecans, oil/dry roasted, 3 ounces
Pork, spare ribs, 3 ounces	Peanut butter, 2 tablespoons	Salmon, canned, pink/red, 3 ounces
Radishes	Pork, boneless loin chop, 3 ounces	Sardines, canned in oil, 3 ounces
Rice cakes, 1 cake	Pork, leg roast, 3 ounces	Scallops, breaded/fried, 3 ounces
Rice, white, enriched, cooked	Raisin Bran, 1 cup	Sole, 3 ounces
Sherbet	Raisins, seedless, 1 cup	Soybeans, mature, boiled
Shrimp, cooked with moist heat, 3 ounces	Rice, brown, cooked, 1 cup	Sunflower seeds, 1 ounce
Sour cream	Shredded Wheat, 1 cup	Swordfish, 3 ounces
Tofu, soft	Shrimp, breaded/fried, 3 ounces	Tofu, raw, firm
Wheat flour, white, 1 cup	Snapper, 3 ounces	Tuna, light, canned in oil, 3 ounces
	Spinach, raw	Tuna, white, canned in oil, 3 ounces
	Tortilla, 2 corn or flour (6-inch diameter)	Veal, cubed, stewed, 3 ounces
	Turkey, breast, 3 ounces	Walnuts, English, 2 ounces
	Turkey, dark meat, 3 ounces	Wheat flour, whole grain, 1 cup
	Veal, rib roast, 3 ounces	Yogurt, low-fat
	Wheat flakes, 1 cup	Yogurt, skim

*One serving = ½ cup unless otherwise noted.

Calories

Calories are present in all foods we eat and give us energy to function every day. Your calorie needs are higher when you have kidney disease, especially if you are on dialysis. If you have stage 3 or 4 chronic kidney disease, you may be advised to make some changes to your diet, especially if you are not at a healthy weight. You may be told to gain or lose a few pounds, depending on your condition. Maintaining a healthy weight can help you control your kidney disease and prevent more health problems. Blood pressure and blood-sugar levels usually improve with a healthy weight-loss regime. In turn, this may delay or prevent more kidney damage.

If you need to add calories to your diet to gain weight, the best way to do this is to add one high-fat food to meals or snacks. Some healthy-fat food options are listed in the "Fats" section of this chapter. In both chronic kidney disease and with dialysis, daily calorie requirements are 30 to 35 calories per kilogram of body weight. So if you weigh 150 pounds, this is about 2,000 calories each day.

Protein

Protein plays a very important role in the body. Your body needs protein to repair tissue, build muscle, and fight infection. That's why eating protein is so crucial to staying healthy. The average person needs between 40 and 65 grams of protein each day. If you're in stages 1, 2, or 3 of chronic kidney disease, your protein intake will be limited to 12 to 15 percent of your calorie intake each day, the same level recommended by the Dietary Reference Intakes (DRIs) for a healthy diet for normal adults. If you're in stage 4 of chronic kidney disease, your protein intake will be reduced to 10 percent of your daily calorie intake.

When dialysis filters out waste from your blood, it also removes protein. That's why it is important you eat enough protein to make up for what is lost. Otherwise, your body will start to use the protein from your muscles to get the protein it needs. This can make you lose weight, feel very tired, and increase your risk of infection. People receiving dialysis should eat about 1.2 grams of protein per kilogram of body weight each day. In other words, if you weigh 150 pounds, this is about 82 grams of protein each day. At least half of the protein you eat should come from high-quality protein sources.

Keeping track of how much protein you eat can help your kidneys work longer. Protein also plays a role in fighting infection and healing wounds, and it provides a source of energy for your body. Here is a list of high-protein foods to make part of your diet.

Common High-Protein Foods*

MEATS, POULTRY, DAIRY, AND EGGS		
Beef, ground, 5% fat	Pollock	Cheese, cottage, creamed
Beef, rib, lean, roasted	Pork, leg, lean, roasted	Cheese, cottage, 2% fat
Beef, bottom round	Pork chops	Cheese, ricotta, part skim milk
Chicken, breast, without skin	Salmon, Atlantic	Cheese, ricotta, whole milk
Chicken, dark meat, without skin	Swordfish	Egg substitute, ¼ cup, 6.0 grams
Cod, Pacific	Tuna, light, canned in oil	Egg whole, 1 large, 6.2 grams
Duck, cooked, without skin	Tuna, yellowfin	Milk, dry, nonfat
Flounder	Tuna salad, 16.5 grams	Yogurt, Greek, plain, nonfat, ⅔ cup, 11 grams
Halibut, Atlantic/Pacific	Veal, rib, lean, roasted	Yogurt, plain, low fat, 13 grams

LEGUMES, NUTS, GRAINS, AND CEREALS		
Almonds, 2 ounces	Lentils, boiled, 1 cup	Bagel (4-inch diameter)
Cashews, dry roasted, 2 ounces	Beans, white, boiled, 1 cup	Bread crumbs, 1 cup
Hazelnuts	Peanuts, dry roasted	Wheat flour, white, 1 cup
Peas, split, boiled, 1 cup	Soybeans, mature, boiled	Wheat flour, whole grain, 1 cup
Pine nuts, dried		
Pistachios, dry roasted		
Walnuts, English, chopped		

*One serving of meat = 3 ounces, providing at least 20 grams of protein unless otherwise noted.
One serving of dairy = 1 cup, providing at least 20 grams of protein unless otherwise noted.
All others, one serving = ½ cup, providing at least 10 grams of protein unless otherwise noted.

Fats

If your blood lipid (fat) levels are high, you may need to cut down on the amount of fat you eat. There is an association between chronic kidney disease and heart disease. An increased risk of heart disease is related to your kidney disease and, typically, to other problems such as diabetes and high blood pressure. It is best to eat healthy fats like olive or canola oil. If your blood potassium and phosphorus levels are low enough to allow it, I would recommend adding avocados, nuts, and seeds to your diet. Tuna and salmon also contain heart-healthy fats that make a good addition to your diet. The key is to keep your fat intake to less than 30 percent of your daily calories. For example, if your calorie allowance is 2,000 calories, your calories from fat should be limited to 600 calories, or about 70 grams of fat.

Sodium

Sodium is a mineral that helps regulate your body's water content and blood pressure. Healthy kidneys can remove sodium from the body as needed, but when your kidneys do not work well, sodium can build up and can cause high blood pressure, fluid-weight gain, and thirst. High blood pressure increases the chance of your kidney disease getting worse. If you are in the early stages of chronic kidney disease (stages 1 to 4), you will need to make some dietary modifications if you have high blood pressure or if you are retaining fluid. If you have stage 5 chronic kidney disease and require dialysis, you will need to follow a low-sodium diet and not consume more than 1,500 milligrams of sodium each day, which is equivalent to a little less than 1 teaspoon of salt. (It is important to note 1 teaspoon of salt each day is the total amount of sodium you are allowed, which includes all foods plus added salt.) Follow a sodium-restricted diet carefully to keep your blood pressure under control. Controlling your blood pressure may also prevent your risk of developing heart disease and decrease the chances of your kidney disease getting worse.

High-Sodium Foods to Avoid

Table salt	Most canned foods	Canned soups
Seasoning salt	Ham	Sauerkraut
Soy sauce	Salt pork	Fast foods
Teriyaki sauce	Microwave meals	Salad dressings
Garlic salt	Potato chips	Hot dogs
Onion salt	Salted crackers	Cold cuts, deli meat
Spam	Buttermilk	Corned beef
Vegetable juices	Canned ravioli	Frozen prepared foods
Barbecue sauce	Bouillon cubes	Bacon
Monosodium glutamate (MSG)		

Low-Sodium Foods to Choose

Fresh garlic	Low-sodium salad dressings	Canned food with no added salt
Fresh onion	Allspice	Low-sodium seasoning blends
Black pepper	Ginger	Fresh fish
Lemon juice	Rosemary	Eggs
Vinegar, regular or flavored	Thyme	Dry mustard
Nuts, unsalted	Dill	Sage
Pretzels, unsalted	Unsalted popcorn	Tarragon
Crackers, unsalted	Homemade broth	

Carbohydrates and Fiber

Some carbohydrate-containing foods also contain fiber, which plays an important role in protecting your heart, blood vessels, and colon. A high-fiber diet will help you lower your fat/cholesterol levels, reducing your risk of a heart attack. When you have kidney disease, you may experience diarrhea and/or constipation. Fiber can help reduce these symptoms plus help control your weight and blood sugar levels. The recommended amount of fiber for people with chronic kidney disease and on dialysis is at least 25 grams per day. This is hard to achieve in a renal diet because of potassium, phosphorus, and fluid restrictions. Don't worry so much about trying to eat a certain number of grams of fiber. Try to add more high-fiber foods that are also renal diet–friendly while staying within your fluid limit. Here is a list of high-fiber foods.

High-Fiber Food Choices*

FRUITS (1–4g fiber)	VEGETABLES (1–4g fiber)	BREADS AND GRAINS (1–6g fiber)
Raspberries, 4.0 grams	Peas, frozen, cooked, 4.0 grams	Barley, pearled, cooked, 6 grams
Blackberries, 4.0 grams	Beans, green/yellow, 3.4 grams	Grape-Nuts Flakes, ¾ cup, 3 grams
Pear, raw with skin, 3.0 grams	Carrots, 1.8 grams	Flaxseed, whole, 1 tablespoon, 2.8 grams
Applesauce, 3 grams	Corn, cooked, 1.8 grams	Rice, brown, cooked, 1.7 grams
Apple, raw with skin, 2.5 grams	Zucchini, cooked, 1 cup, 1.8 grams	Bread, white, 2 slices, 1.6 grams
Blueberries, 1.8 grams	Asparagus, 1.4 grams	Air-popped popcorn, 1 cup, 1.2 grams
Tangerine, 1.8 grams	Cabbage, raw, 1.1 grams	Corn grits, yellow, cooked, 1 cup, 1.0 gram
Strawberries, sliced, 1.7 grams	Broccoli, 1.1 grams	Cornflakes, 1 cup, 1.0 gram
Apricot, halves, 1.5 grams	Cauliflower, cooked, 1.0 gram	

*One serving = ½ cup unless otherwise noted.

WHOLE GRAINS: THE WHOLE STORY

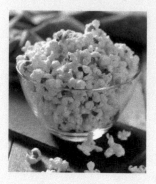

You've probably heard of whole grains, but you aren't quite sure what they really are. They are grains that have not been processed and include all original nutrients. In whole grains, endosperm, bran, and germ are left intact. Whole grains are rich in fiber, vitamins, iron, magnesium, and selenium.

Whole grains have been typically restricted for those with kidney disease because they also contain phosphorus and potassium, which typically need to be limited. However, depending on your blood phosphorus and potassium levels, whole grains in moderation can be very beneficial.

The health benefits of whole grains include improved digestive health, lowered cholesterol levels, and lowered risk of heart disease and stroke. Whole grains contain fiber, and fiber also aids in cancer prevention.

Whole grains with lower potassium and phosphorus content:

Barley

Buckwheat

Bulgur

Popcorn

Wild rice

Whole grains with higher potassium and phosphorus content:

Amaranth

Brown rice

Millet

Oats

Quinoa

Spelt

Vitamin and Mineral Supplements

If you have kidney disease or you are receiving dialysis, over-the-counter multivitamins may not be good for your health. Vitamins A, E, and K must be limited or even avoided, because levels of these vitamins build up in the body as kidney function decreases. Some multivitamins do not have enough water-soluble vitamins, such as B-complex and folic acid. These kinds of vitamins do not build up in the body and must be replaced daily, so you need more of them. Talk with your physician about getting a prescription for a renal multivitamin.

Fluids

Depending on your stage of kidney disease, you may need to limit the fluids you drink. Fluid is any food or beverage that turns to liquid at room temperature. It includes water and ice cubes; tea; coffee; juice; soft drinks; milk and milk products; gravy, sauces, and soups; ice cream; jelly and gelatin; custard; and yogurt.

Drinking too much fluid can result in fluid retention. This can lead to increased blood pressure and edema (swelling), and it may cause congestive heart failure. In the early stages of chronic kidney disease, you can drink your normal amount of fluid. In the later stages and when you receive dialysis, your suggested fluid intake will depend on your urine output, fluid buildup, and blood pressure. When you are receiving dialysis, liquids are usually limited to 32 to 48 ounces, or 1,000 to 1,500 milliliters, each day.

"Double Trouble" Foods

Following a renal diet can be a little tricky because some foods that are high in potassium are also high in phosphorus. Double trouble foods—those that are high in both potassium and phosphorus—include milk and dairy foods, nuts, seeds, chocolate, and whole-grain products. These are foods that are best to avoid or use in very small amounts. This table was created to help improve your chances of keeping your potassium and phosphorus level under control.

How to Avoid "Double Trouble" Foods

INSTEAD OF THESE...	TRY THESE...
Cheese	Low-fat cottage cheese, 1 ounce of cream cheese or hard cheese, sprinkle of Parmesan cheese
Cream soup	Broth-based soups made with puréed vegetables
Dried beans or peas	Green beans and wax greens
Ice cream	Sorbet, ice pops, sherbet, Tofutti frozen desserts
Milk, coconut milk	Almond milk, rice milk, Rich's Coffee Rich, Rice Dream Original
Nuts, low-salt snack foods	Pretzels, tortilla chips, popcorn, crackers
Peanut butter, nut butter, and Nutella	Low-fat cream cheese, jam or fruit spread

NO MEAT? NO PROBLEM.

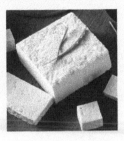 A vegetarian is someone who doesn't eat meat and mostly eats foods that come from plants, such as grains, fruits, vegetables, and nuts. Whether you are lacto-ovo vegetarian or vegan, your food choices can be adapted to a diet designed for kidney-disease management.

Vegetarians can be classified into four categories:

Lacto-vegetarians: People who eat dairy products and plant foods but exclude eggs and meat

Lacto-ovo vegetarians: People who eat eggs, dairy products, and plant foods, but no meats

Pesco-vegetarians: People who eat fish in addition to eating plant foods, dairy products, and eggs

Vegans: People who only eat plant foods and no animal products

Below are the some of the best sources of high-quality plant proteins, including choices for vegetarians who follow a lacto-ovo diet. Choose three or more different protein choices each day. Soy protein is a good choice for vegetarians; it is best to include at least one soy item in your diet daily. Some of the recommendations contain phosphorus and potassium, so the following suggestions are only for people who eat a plant-based diet and do not consume any meat.

Good sources of protein for vegetarians following a renal-friendly diet include the following:

Dairy products
Eggs and egg substitutes
Grains
Lentils

Meat substitutes: soy burgers, soy-based low-sodium hot dogs and deli slices
Seitan
Soy products: tofu, tempeh
Unsalted natto (fermented soybeans)

CHAPTER THREE

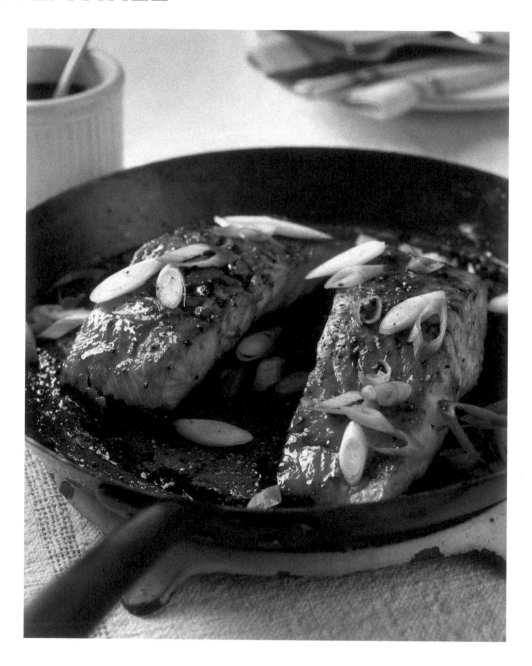

MEAL PLAN IN ACTION

Watching what you eat and drink is very important when you have chronic kidney disease. The 28-day meal plan I designed for this book is not only kidney friendly but is also aimed at helping you stay with your dietary changes over the long term. The recipes are part of the meal plan and can be enjoyed any day to spark some creativity with your diet. These meal plans are created to help you stay on track, save you money, cook with ease, save time, and reduce waste.

Preparing for the Diet

Before you get to enjoy the benefits that come with following a renal diet, you first must undergo a mental makeover to break old, bad habits. The key to beginning the diet is thinking of it properly—as a true lifestyle change instead of a hard-to-follow renal diet. Think of your goal as a healthier lifestyle, and remember that you want to stick to your renal diet for the foreseeable future.

Now that you have a positive attitude, the next step is to give your pantry a makeover. Clean out your fridge and throw out expired food in your refrigerator and pantry. Next, toss out (or donate to your local food pantry) the empty-calorie foods with little nutritional value, including soda, sweetened drinks, packaged sweets, chips, and dessert mixes. Don't feel pressured to deprive yourself of every indulgence; everything can be eaten in moderation. But make sure the junk foods do not make up a large portion of your pantry.

Lastly, set aside some time to make a grocery list and to concentrate on grocery shopping. A grocery list is an essential part of shopping and helps eliminate the guesswork. Without a list, you will tend to buy many things you don't need and spend a lot more money. Spending an adequate amount of time at the grocery store instead of rushing will allow you time to read the ingredient lists and nutrition labels.

Shopping Tips

Reading food labels is essential to making healthy food choices for your kidneys. When you have chronic kidney disease, you may need to limit some minerals and nutrients in your diet, such as sodium, phosphorus, and potassium. The amount of fat you eat should also be limited, especially saturated fats and trans fats. The Nutrition Facts label will serve as a guide to help you make healthier choices. Here are some words to look for when reading the Nutrition Facts label:

- Claims such as "low in saturated fat" or "fat-free"

- "No salt-added," "sodium-free," "sodium-restricted," and "unsalted"

Nutrition Facts

Serving Size ¼ cup (50g)
Servings per Container 18

Amount Per Serving

Calories 300	Calories from Fat 110

	% Daily Value
Total Fat 12g	20%
Saturated Fat 4g	22%
Cholesterol 0mg	0%
Sodium 200 mg	8%
Total Carbohydrate 30g	10%
Dietary Fiber 0g	0%
Sugars 20g	
Protein 5g	

Vitamin A 5%	Vitamin C 0%
Calcium 10%	Iron 0%

* Percent Daily Values are based on a 2,000 calorie diet.

The amount listed is for ¼ cup serving. If you eat ½ cup, you've eaten two servings.

One serving has 200 milligrams of sodium.

This package has 18 servings; each serving is ¼ cup.

One serving has 8% of the daily value of sodium.

140 milligrams or less per serving is considered low sodium.

TOOLS FOR SUCCESS

You don't need a lot of kitchen gadgets to help with meal preparation, but investing in a good chef's knife will make the process easier and safer and having nonstick cookware on hand will keep the meals low-fat so you don't have to use additional butter or oil to prevent food from sticking to the pan.

Check the ingredient list for phosphorus or for words that start with "phos." Many packaged goods contain phosphorus. It may be best to choose a different food item when the ingredient list has "phos" in the nutrition label. Here is an example for potato chips:

> **Ingredients:** potatoes, modified cornstarch, lactic acid, disodium phosphate, citric acid, calcium lactate.

Check the ingredient list for potassium. For example, potassium chloride can be added in place of salt in some packaged goods, like canned soups and tomato products. It is best to limit these foods with potassium on the ingredient list. Here is an example for tomato juice:

> **Ingredients:** reconstituted vegetable juice blend, water, contains less than 2% of: potassium chloride, magnesium, salt, natural flavoring, vitamin C (ascorbic acid), citric acid.

Stocking a Kidney-Friendly Pantry

A well-stocked kitchen will ensure you have everything you need to cook and enjoy kidney-friendly meals, all while helping you feel better. Having healthy ingredients and snacks in your pantry and refrigerator will give you kidney-friendly nourishment all day long.

On the following pages are some items that will help you create your grocery list for your next trip to the store. You don't have to buy everything on the list; rather, use this list as a guide for your kitchen staples. This list will help you find kidney-friendly goods at the grocery store that you can stock up on every month. People with diabetes will want to be cautious of sugar intake when looking at the beverages and sweets sections.

Grocery List for a Kidney-Friendly Pantry

Meat and Meat Substitutes

Beef	Fish	Tuna, canned
Chicken	Lamb	Turkey
Eggs	Pork, chops/ roast	Veal
Egg substitute	Tofu	

Vegetables

Alfalfa sprouts	Chiles	Lettuce
Arugula	Chives	Onions
Asparagus	Coleslaw	Parsley
Bean sprouts	Corn	Radishes
Beets, canned	Cucumber	Spaghetti squash
Cabbage, green/red	Eggplant	Turnips
Carrots	Endive	Vegetables, mixed
Cauliflower	Ginger root	Water chestnuts, canned
Celery	Green beans	

Fruits

Apple juice	Cranberry sauce	Peach nectar
Apples	Figs, fresh	Pear nectar
Applesauce	Fruit cocktail	Pears, canned
Apricot nectar	Grapefruit	Pineapple
Apricots, canned	Grapefruit juice	Plums
Blackberries	Grapes	Raspberries
Cherries	Lemon	Strawberries
Cranberries	Lime	Tangerines
Cranberry juice	Peaches	Watermelon

Breads and Cereals

Bagels, plain/blueberry	Cereals, Kellogg's Corn Flakes	Cereals, Corn Chex
Bread, white/French/ Italian	Cereals, Cheerios	Couscous
		Crackers, unsalted

Dinner rolls

English muffins

Grits

Hamburger/
  hot dog rolls

Pasta

Melba toast

Noodles

Oyster crackers

Pita bread

Pretzels, unsalted

Rice, brown/white

Spaghetti

Tortillas

Fats

Butter

Canola oil

Cream cheese

Margarine

Mayonnaise

Miracle Whip

Nondairy creamers

Olive oil

Sweets

Animal crackers

Angel food cake

Candy corn

Chewing gum

Cotton candy

Crispy rice treats

Graham crackers

Gumdrops

Gummy bears

Hard candy

Hot Tamales candy

Jell-O

Jelly beans

Jolly Rancher

Lemon cake

Life Savers

Marshmallows

Newtons (fig, strawberry,
  apple, blueberry)

Pie (apple, berry, cherry,
  lemon, peach)

Pound cake

Rice cakes

Vanilla wafers

Beverages

7UP

Coffee

Cream soda

Fruit punch

Ginger ale

Grape soda

Hi-C

Lemon-lime soda

Lemonade

Orange soda

Root beer

Tea

Dairy and Dairy Alternatives

Almond milk

Coffee-mate

Mocha Mix

Rice Dream

Rich's Coffee Rich

Other

Apple butter

Corn syrup

Honey

Jam

Jelly

Maple syrup

Sugar, brown or white

Sugar, powdered

TIME-SAVING STRATEGIES

If you are always on the go, with errands to run, dinner to make, and a schedule to maintain, grocery shopping can test your patience. Maintaining a healthy, appropriate diet comes down to effective meal planning and grocery shopping. While many people who don't have chronic kidney disease may buy food at random during the week, people with kidney disease need to do a bit more planning and have an effective grocery-store strategy.

Keep yourself on track with these six tips for efficient food shopping:

1. Don't shop on an empty stomach. Go shopping after you've eaten. This will help you avoid buying unhealthy food products.

2. Have your shopping list ready. Keep your grocery list organized and efficient, arranging items by category or grouping items that are usually found in the same aisle. There are two advantages to this trick: you spend less time in the grocery store, and you are less likely to forget something.

3. Plan ahead. Try to plan out your meals and foods for the week. It will save you time, and you won't stress out over daily menu planning.

4. Keep it simple. Your shopping trip doesn't have to be time-consuming. Do you have coffee, sugar, cereal, bread, fruit, or milk? What will you be packing for lunch? Do you have the recipe, so you can jot down the ingredients you need ahead of time?

5. Stick to the list. When you go to the grocery store, do not stray from your list. Avoid impulse buys because this will help you avoid unhealthy purchases and save you money.

6. Fresh is best. One of the best places to grocery shop is at your local farmers' market. Farmers' markets always have the freshest and most delicious produce. When you consider the value of organic, local foods and their potential positive effect on your health, you won't mind paying a little more at the farmers' market.

Eating healthy and maintaining a diet that's kidney-friendly doesn't have to be hard. With the right amount of planning, a little prep work, and a good grocery-store strategy, creating a healthy meal plan can be easy and fun.

28-DAY MEAL PLAN

This 28-day meal plan is designed to take some of the guesswork out of planning your meals and shopping for ingredients. The shopping lists include everything you need for making breakfast, lunch, and dinner for the week, but note that ingredients for snacks are not listed. Once you decide which snacks you wish to have on hand, you can include those ingredients. Some items on the shopping lists might already be in your pantry, so take a look at the quantities needed for the week and buy an ingredient only if you need it.

If you make a pot of chicken stock in the first week, you can freeze it in 1-cup quantities to use for the rest of the meal plan. If you have leftovers from any meal, substitute them into the meal plan as a snack or another meal later in the week. The protein intake for each day ranges between 35 and 50 grams, so if you need more protein in your diet, include high-protein snacks or increase the portion sizes of high-protein dishes. When in doubt, consult a registered dietitian to ensure your specific needs are met.

Week 1 Meal Plan

THE
28-DAY
MEAL
PLAN:
WEEK 1

Monday:

Breakfast: Mixed-Grain Hot Cereal

Lunch: Traditional Chicken-Vegetable Soup

Dinner: Baked Cod with Cucumber-Dill Salsa

Tuesday:

Breakfast: Corn Pudding

Lunch: Crab Cakes with Lime Salsa

Dinner: Pesto Pork Chops

Wednesday:

Breakfast: Fruit and Cheese Breakfast Wrap

Lunch: Linguine with Roasted Red Pepper–Basil Sauce

Dinner: Herb Pesto Tuna

Thursday:

Breakfast: Cinnamon-Nutmeg Blueberry Muffins

Lunch: Egg White Frittata with Penne

Dinner: Lemon-Herb Chicken

Friday:

Breakfast: Egg-in-the-Hole

Lunch: Five-Spice Chicken Lettuce Wraps

Dinner: Sweet Glazed Salmon

Saturday:

Breakfast: Skillet-Baked Pancake

Lunch: Turkey-Bulgur Soup

Dinner: Grilled Steak with Cucumber-Cilantro Salsa

Sunday:

Breakfast: Strawberry–Cream Cheese Stuffed French Toast

Lunch: Couscous Burgers

Dinner: Indian Chicken Curry

Suggested Snacks:

Cinnamon Applesauce (page 79)

Blueberry-Pineapple Smoothie (page 103)

Spicy Kale Chips (page 126)

Hard-boiled eggs

Grapes

Ice pops

Rice cakes

Week 1 Shopping List

Fruits and Vegetables

Apples (2)

Blueberries (8 ounces)

Cabbage, green, shredded (½ cup)

Carrots (4)

Celery stalks (7)

Corn, frozen kernels (2 cups)

Cucumbers, English (2)

Garlic (16 cloves, or 9 teaspoons minced
   and 4 cloves)

Jalapeño pepper (1)

Lemons (4)

Lettuce, Boston (1 head)

Limes (4)

Onions, sweet (5)

Peppers, bell, red (2)

Scallions (4)

Snow peas (½ cup)

Sprouts, bean (½ cup)

Dairy and Dairy Alternatives

Butter, unsalted (¾ cup)

Cheese, cream, plain (5 ounces)

Cheese, Parmesan, low-fat (1 ounce)

Eggs (18 eggs)

Milk, coconut (¼ cup)

Milk, unsweetened rice (4½ cups)

Milk, vanilla, rice, not enriched
   (1¼ cups)

Sour cream, light (2 tablespoons)

Spices and Herbs

Basil, fresh (2 bunches)

Bay leaves, dried (4)

Cardamon, ground

Cayenne pepper

Chinese five-spice powder

Chives, fresh (1 bunch)

Cilantro, fresh (1 bunch)

Cinnamon, ground

Cloves, ground

Coriander, ground

Cumin, ground

Curry powder

Dill, fresh (1 bunch)

Fennel powder

Ginger, fresh (2-inch piece)

Ginger, ground

Green chili powder

Mustard, ground

Nutmeg, ground

Oregano, fresh (1 bunch)

Parsley, fresh (1 bunch)

Peppercorns, black,
   freshly ground

Peppercorns, black

Red pepper flakes

Sage, fresh (1 bunch)

Sweet paprika, ground

Thyme, fresh (1 bunch)

Turmeric, ground

▶

Week 1 Shopping List continued

Fish and Seafood

Cod (4 fillets totaling 12 ounces)

Crab meat, queen (8 ounces)

Salmon (4 fillets totaling 12 ounces)

Shrimp (8 ounces)

Tuna, yellowfin (4 fillets totaling
   12 ounces)

Meat and Poultry

Beef, tenderloin (4 steaks totaling
   12 ounces)

Chicken breasts, boneless, skinless
   (36 ounces)

Chicken carcass, skin removed (1)

Chicken thighs, boneless, skinless (6)

Pork, top loin (4 chops totaling
   12 ounces)

Turkey, ground, 93% lean (8 ounces)

Other

Baking soda substitute, Ener-G
   (3½ teaspoons)

Bread, Italian (2 slices)

Bread, white (8 slices)

Bread crumbs

Buckwheat, whole (2 tablespoons)

Bulgur (½ cup)

Chickpeas (4 ounces)

Cooking spray

Couscous (2 cups)

Flour, all-purpose

Honey

Hot pepper sauce

Jam, strawberry (¼ cup)

Linguine

Oil, canola

Oil, olive

Penne

Sugar, granulated

Tortillas, flour, 6-inch diameter (2)

Vanilla extract, pure

Vinegar, apple cider

Vinegar, balsamic

Week 2 Meal Plan

Monday:

Breakfast: Fruit and Cheese
  Breakfast Wrap

Lunch: Indian Chicken Curry

Dinner: Classic Pot Roast

Tuesday:

Breakfast: Mixed-Grain Hot Cereal

Lunch: Roasted Beef Stew

Dinner: Sweet Glazed Salmon

Wednesday:

Breakfast: Cinnamon-Nutmeg
  Blueberry Muffins

Lunch: Couscous Burgers

Dinner: Persian Chicken

Thursday:

Breakfast: Egg-in-the-Hole

Lunch: Five-Spice Chicken
  Lettuce Wraps

Dinner: Baked Cod with Cucumber-
  Dill Salsa

Friday:

Breakfast: Corn Pudding

Lunch: Traditional Chicken-
  Vegetable Soup

Dinner: Sweet and Sour Meat Loaf

Saturday:

Breakfast: Strawberry–Cream Cheese
  Stuffed French Toast

Lunch: Egg White Frittata with Penne

Dinner: Pesto Pork Chops

Sunday:

Breakfast: Skillet-Baked Pancake

Lunch: Linguine with Roasted Red
  Pepper–Basil Sauce

Dinner: Herb Pesto Tuna

Suggested Snacks:

Cooked Four-Pepper Salsa with
  baked pita wedges (page 76)

Apple-Chai Smoothie (page 102)

Meringue Cookies (page 131)

Tuna salad

Apple

Unsalted popcorn

Watermelon

THE
28-DAY
MEAL
PLAN:
WEEK 2

Week 2 Shopping List

THE 28-DAY MEAL PLAN: WEEK 2

Fruits and Vegetables

Apples (2)

Blueberries (8 ounces)

Carrots (4)

Celery stalks (8)

Corn, frozen kernels (2 cups)

Cucumber, English (1)

Garlic (14 cloves or 10 teaspoons minced and 2 cloves)

Lemons (4)

Lettuce, Boston (1 head)

Limes (2)

Onions, sweet (6)

Peppers, banana (2)

Peppers, bell, red (2)

Pepper, bell, green (1)

Pepper, jalapeño (2)

Scallion (2)

Snow peas (½ cup)

Sprouts, bean (½ cup)

Dairy and Dairy Alternatives

Butter, unsalted (½ cup)

Cheese, Parmesan, low-fat (1 ounce)

Cheese, cream, plain (5 ounces)

Eggs (18)

Sour cream, light (2 tablespoons)

Milk, coconut (¼ cup)

Milk, rice, unsweetened (4 cups)

Milk, rice, vanilla (1¼ cups)

Spices and Herbs

Basil, fresh (1 bunch)

Bay leaves (2)

Black pepper

Cardamom, ground

Cayenne pepper

Chinese five-spice powder

Chives, fresh (1 bunch)

Cilantro, fresh (1 bunch)

Cinnamon, ground

Cloves, ground

Coriander, ground

Cumin, ground

Dill, fresh (1 bunch)

Fennel powder

Garlic powder

Ginger, fresh (2 teaspoons)

Ginger, ground

Green chili powder

Mustard, ground

Nutmeg, ground

Oregano, dried

Oregano, fresh (1 bunch)

Paprika, sweet

Parsley, fresh (1 bunch)

Peppercorns, black

Red pepper flakes

Thyme, dried

Thyme, fresh (1 bunch)

Turmeric, ground

Fish and Seafood

Cod (4 fillets totaling 12 ounces)

Salmon (4 fillets totaling 12 ounces)

Shrimp (8 ounces)

Tuna, yellowfin (4 fillets totaling
12 ounces)

Meat and Poultry

Beef, ground, 95% lean (1 pound)

Beef, roast, chuck or rump
(1½ pounds, divided into
1 pound and ½ pound)

Chicken carcass (1)

Chicken breasts, boneless, skinless
(24 ounces, or family pack)

Chicken thighs, boneless,
skinless (11)

Pork, top loin (4 chops totaling
12 ounces)

Other

Baking soda substitute, Ener-G
(1½ teaspoons)

Beef stock (1 cup)

Bread crumbs

Bread, Italian (2 slices)

Bread, white (8 slices)

Buckwheat, whole (2 tablespoons)

Bulgur (6 tablespoons)

Chickpeas, canned (4 ounces)

Cooking spray

Cornstarch

Couscous (2½ cups plus
6 tablespoons)

Flour, all-purpose

Honey

Jam, strawberry (¼ cup)

Linguine

Oil, canola

Oil, olive

Penne

Sugar, brown

Sugar, granulated

Tortillas, flour, 6-inch diameter (2)

Vanilla extract, pure

Vinegar, apple cider

Vinegar, balsamic

Vinegar, white

Week 3 Meal Plan

Monday:

Breakfast: Cheesy Scrambled Eggs with Fresh Herbs

Lunch: Couscous Burgers

Dinner: Indian Chicken Curry (leftover)

Tuesday:

Breakfast: Mixed-Grain Hot Cereal

Lunch: Crab Cakes with Lime Salsa

Dinner: Sweet and Sour Meat Loaf

Wednesday:

Breakfast: Corn Pudding

Lunch: Sweet and Sour Meat Loaf (leftover)

Dinner: Persian Chicken

Thursday:

Breakfast: Cinnamon-Nutmeg Blueberry Muffins

Lunch: Ginger Beef Salad

Dinner: Herb Pesto Tuna

Friday:

Breakfast: Fruit and Cheese Breakfast Wrap

Lunch: Roasted Beef Stew

Dinner: Lemon-Herb Chicken

Saturday:

Breakfast: Curried Egg Pita Pockets

Lunch: Turkey-Bulgur Soup

Dinner: Grilled Steak with Cucumber-Cilantro Salsa

Sunday:

Breakfast: Strawberry–Cream Cheese Stuffed French Toast

Lunch: Egg White Frittata with Penne

Dinner: Baked Cod with Cucumber-Dill Salsa

Suggested Snacks:

Cinnamon Applesauce (page 79)

Festive Berry Parfait (page 105)

Corn Bread (page 132)

Tuna salad

Cucumber sticks

Mixed berries

Graham crackers

Week 3 Shopping List

Fruits and Vegetables

Apples (2)

Blueberries (8 ounces)

Cabbage, green, shredded (½ cup)

Carrots (2)

Celery stalks (3)

Corn, frozen kernels (2 cups)

Cucumbers, English (2)

Garlic (14 cloves or 10 teaspoons
    minced garlic and 2 cloves)

Lemons (6)

Lettuce, leaf, green (1 head)

Limes (5)

Onion, red (1)

Onions, sweet (2)

Peppers, bell, red (3)

Scallions (4)

Watercress (1 bunch)

Dairy and Dairy Alternatives

Butter, unsalted (¾ cup)

Cheese, cream, plain (10 ounces)

Eggs (24)

Milk, coconut (¼ cup)

Milk, rice, unsweetened (4 cups)

Milk, rice, vanilla (1¼ cups)

Sour cream, light (4 tablespoons)

Spices and Herbs

Basil, fresh (1 bunch)

Bay leaves, dried (2)

Cayenne pepper

Chives, fresh (1 bunch)

Cilantro, fresh (1 bunch)

Cinnamon, ground

Cumin, ground

Curry powder

Dill, fresh (1 bunch)

Garlic powder

Ginger, fresh (4-inch piece)

Ginger, ground

Green chili powder

Nutmeg, ground

Oregano, dried

Oregano, fresh (1 bunch)

Paprika, sweet

Parsley, fresh (1 bunch)

Peppercorns, black, freshly ground

Red pepper flakes

Sage, fresh (1 bunch)

Tarragon, fresh (1 bunch)

Thyme, fresh (1 bunch)

Fish and Seafood

Cod (4 fillets totaling 12 ounces)

Crab meat, queen (8 ounces)

Tuna, yellowfin (4 fillets totaling
    12 ounces)

▶

Week 3 Shopping List *continued*

THE
28-DAY
MEAL
PLAN:
WEEK 3

Meat and Poultry

Beef, ground, 95% lean (1 pound)

Beef, roast, chuck (½ pound)

Beef, steak, flank (¾ pound)

Beef, tenderloin (4 steaks totaling
   12 ounces)

Chicken breasts, boneless, skinless
   (12 ounces)

Chicken thighs, boneless, skinless (11)

Pork, top loin (4 chops totaling
   12 ounces)

Turkey, ground, 93% lean (5 ounces)

Other

Baking soda substitute, Ener-G
   (3½ teaspoons)

Bread crumbs

Bread, pita pockets,
   4-inch diameter (2)

Bread, white (8 slices)

Buckwheat, whole (2 tablespoons)

Bulgur (1 cup)

Chickpeas (4 ounces)

Chili paste (1 teaspoon)

Cooking spray

Cornstarch

Couscous (3 cups)

Flour, all-purpose

Honey

Hot pepper sauce

Jam, strawberry (¼ cup)

Oil, canola

Oil, olive

Penne

Stock, beef (1 cup)

Sugar, brown

Sugar, granulated

Tortillas, flour, 6-inch diameter (2)

Vanilla extract, pure

Vinegar, apple cider

Vinegar, white

Week 4 Meal Plan

Monday:

Breakfast: Egg-in-the-Hole

Lunch: Crab Cakes with Lime Salsa

Dinner: Pesto Pork Chops

Tuesday:

Breakfast: Corn Pudding

Lunch: Five-Spice Chicken Lettuce Wraps

Dinner: Sweet Glazed Salmon

Wednesday:

Breakfast: Fruit and Cheese Breakfast Wrap

Lunch: Egg White Frittata with Penne

Dinner: Indian Chicken Curry

Thursday:

Breakfast: Rhubarb Bread Pudding

Lunch: Indian Chicken Curry

Dinner: Couscous Burgers

Friday:

Breakfast: Mixed-Grain Hot Cereal

Lunch: Traditional Chicken-Vegetable Soup

Dinner: Grilled Steak with Cucumber-Cilantro Salsa

Saturday:

Breakfast: Skillet-Baked Pancake

Lunch: Linguine with Roasted Red Pepper–Basil Sauce

Dinner: Herb Pesto Tuna

Sunday:

Breakfast: Cheesy Scrambled Eggs with Fresh Herbs

Lunch: Roasted Beef Stew

Dinner: Lemon-Herb Chicken

Suggested Snacks:

Cinnamon Applesauce (page 79)

Blueberry-Pineapple Smoothie (page 103)

Roasted Red Pepper and Chicken Crostini (page 133)

Deviled eggs

Grapes

Vanilla wafer cookies

Carrot sticks

Week 4 Shopping List

Fruits and Vegetables

Apples (2)

Carrots (2)

Celery stalks (4)

Corn, frozen kernels (2 cups)

Cucumber, English (1)

Garlic (14 cloves or 10 teaspoons
   minced garlic and 2 cloves)

Lemons (4)

Lettuce, Boston (1 head)

Limes (3)

Onions, sweet (4)

Peppers, red, bell (2)

Rhubarb (6 stalks)

Scallions (4)

Sprouts, bean (½ cup)

Dairy and Dairy Alternatives

Butter, unsalted (¾ cup)

Cheese, cream, plain (5 ounces)

Cheese, Parmesan, low-fat (1 ounce)

Eggs (25)

Milk, coconut (¼ cup)

Milk, rice, unsweetened (3¼ cups)

Milk, rice, vanilla (1¼ cups)

Sour cream, light (2 tablespoons)

Spices and Herbs

Basil, fresh (1 bunch)

Cayenne pepper

Chinese five-spice powder

Chives, fresh (1 bunch)

Cilantro, fresh (1 bunch)

Cinnamon, ground

Curry powder

Ginger, fresh (2-inch piece)

Green chili powder

Nutmeg, ground

Oregano, fresh (1 bunch)

Parsley, fresh (1 bunch)

Pepper, black, freshly ground

Red pepper flakes

Tarragon, fresh (1 bunch)

Thyme, fresh (1 bunch)

Vanilla bean (1)

Fish and Seafood

Crab meat, queen (8 ounces)

Salmon (4 fillets totaling 12 ounces)

Tuna, yellowfin (4 fillets totaling
12 ounces)

Meat and Poultry

Beef, roast, chuck (½ pound)

Beef, tenderloin (4 steaks totaling
12 ounces)

Chicken breasts, boneless, skinless
(32 ounces, or family pack)

Chicken thighs, boneless, skinless (6)

Pork, chops, top loin (4 chops totaling
12 ounces)

Other

Baking soda substitute, Ener-G
(½ teaspoon)

Bread crumbs

Bread, Italian (1 loaf)

Bread, white (10 slices)

Buckwheat, whole (2 tablespoons)

Bulgur (6 tablespoons)

Chickpeas (4 ounces)

Cooking spray

Cornstarch

Couscous (2 cups)

Flour, all-purpose

Honey

Hot pepper sauce

Oil, olive

Penne

Spaghetti

Stock, beef (1 cup)

Sugar, granulated

Tortillas, flour, 6-inch diameter (2)

Vinegar, balsamic

CHAPTER FOUR

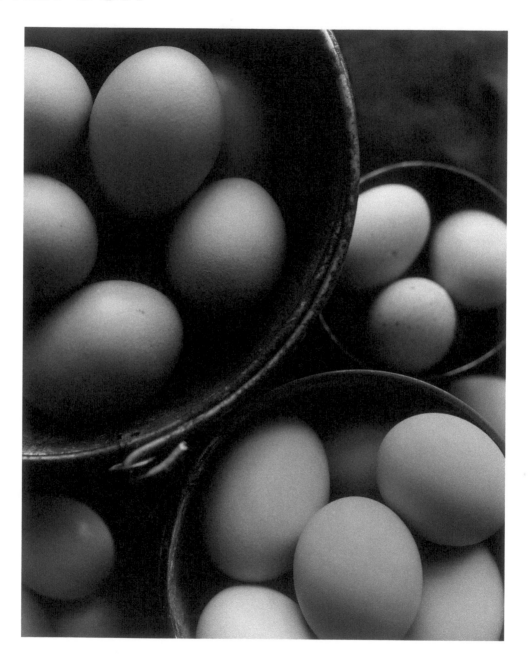

LIVING ON A KIDNEY-HEALTHY DIET

By now, you've probably realized that the kidney-healthy diet isn't a "diet" after all. The 28-day meal plan is designed to help you kick-start your journey to better health with respect to your kidney function. Maintaining this diet after the 28-day meal plan will only get easier from here. Beyond the recipes for the meal plans, I've also included kidney-healthy recipes that you may want to try. You can also experiment with the recipes you may want to make again, some of which may become staples in your diet. Chapter six, Spice Blends and Seasonings, explains how you can add homemade seasonings, rubs, and mixes to certain dishes, particularly dishes featuring protein. It is important to plan your meals with the right amount of protein and calories while adding variety and keeping your potassium, phosphorus, and sodium intake in acceptable amounts.

Handling the Cravings

Once in a while, we all like to treat ourselves to a few goodies, and that's okay. But let's not forget that high-sugar food items, such as cakes, cookies, and chips, offer empty calories with little or no nutritional value. There are many easy-to-make, delicious recipes included in this book that will satisfy your sweet tooth. Make sure to keep gelatin, hard candies, ice pops, sherbet, and vanilla wafers in your pantry to help you stay on track. Occasionally, allow yourself to have a scoop of ice cream or a slice of vanilla cake. If you eat in moderation and make better choices that are compatible with your kidney-heath needs, you can enjoy these sweets without complications.

Low-Sodium Seasoning Choices

Controlling sodium intake is important for those with chronic kidney disease, but a low-sodium renal diet doesn't mean your meals have to be bland. With a little creativity and experimentation with a variety of herbs and spices, your meals can be quite enjoyable. Popular herbs and spices you can use when cooking beef, pork, chicken, fish, and vegetables include allspice, bay leaf, black pepper, caraway, cardamom, curry, dill, fresh garlic, fresh onion, ginger, lemon juice, marjoram, rosemary, thyme, sage, and tarragon.

There also are salt-free blends you can purchase, including Mrs. Dash seasoning blends, Lawry's Salt-Free 17 Seasoning, Chef Paul Prudhomme's Magic Salt-Free Seasonings, and Bragg Organic Sprinkle 24 Herbs and Spices Seasoning. Always check the ingredient list of any seasoning mix to avoid blends with salt and potassium. A great option is to make your own seasoning mixes. There are 16 unique recipes outlined in chapter six, Spice Blends and Seasonings. As you'll see, they are easier to make than you may think!

KIDNEY-FRIENDLY BEVERAGES

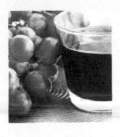

Depending on what stage of kidney disease you are in, you may need to monitor what you drink. Several types of beverages, especially many of the dark sodas, have a lot of phosphate and potassium additives. Aside from what you eat, what you drink also plays an important role in a kidney-friendly diet. You can still enjoy a variety of acceptable drinks, like apple juice, grape juice and cranberry juice. Fresh-brewed coffee and tea (in moderation), water, lemonade, fruit drinks, and bottled teas without additives are also better choices. It is critical to check the ingredient labels of bottled or canned drinks for potassium or phosphate additives.

Dining Out

Dining out can still be an enjoyable experience even on a renal diet. It's all about making smart meal choices and picking foods that are low in sodium, phosphorus, and potassium. The table on the following pages lists some guidelines that will help you make better choices when you're out enjoying your favorite type of cuisine.

Make sure to have a good plan in place when dining out. When in doubt, go online and view the menu, if available, before you visit a restaurant. Prepare any questions you may have for the server. In today's very health-conscious age, restaurant personnel are used to special requests for foods items and preparations.

Be mindful of portion sizes. An easy way to limit your sodium, phosphorus, and potassium intake is to share your meal. Or eat half of your meal at the restaurant and take the other half home, because restaurant portions are often too big.

Strategies for Dining Out

TYPE OF FOOD	AVOID/LIMIT	BETTER CHOICES
Buffet	Soups (generally high in sodium and potassium); chips, potato wedges, roasted or baked potatoes; raw spinach; olives; pickles; bacon bits; tomatoes; mushrooms; broccoli; kidney beans; seeds or nuts; croutons; potato salad; three-bean salad; olive salads; relishes; pickles; dried fruit; fresh fruit salad; kiwi; melons; bananas; oranges	Salad bar (limit serving size to that of a bread and butter plate or a small bowl): lettuce, carrots, radishes, cauliflower, green peppers, celery, onions, cucumbers, green peas, beets, alfalfa sprouts, Chinese noodles, grated cheese (in moderation), coleslaw, macaroni salad, gelatin salads, cottage cheese, canned peaches or pears, canned fruit cocktail, fresh grapes, fresh or canned pineapple, small fresh peach

Grilled, pan-fried, or marinated meats; chicken; fish; seafood |
| Asian | Nuts; green leafy vegetables such as bok choy, Chinese spinach, and Chinese cabbage; fried rice; soy sauce; teriyaki sauce | Egg rolls, dim sum, pot stickers

Steamed veggies, rice, plain noodles (lower-fat choices)

Request that your food be prepared without soy sauce, fish sauce, or monosodium glutamate (MSG), all of which contain a lot of salt |
| Fast Food | French fries (high in potassium), fried fish, fried chicken, ketchup, mustard, milkshakes, dark sodas | Unsalted onion rings (as a substitute for French fries)

Salads, when available

Ask that condiments be left on the side

Burger King: plain hamburger

McDonalds: plain hamburger

Taco Bell: taco with few or no tomatoes

Wendy's: plain single hamburger or grilled chicken sandwich |
| Mexican | Beans, guacamole, cheese, tomatoes | Plain rice, tacos, burritos, fajitas, and enchiladas filled with minced meat, beef, or chicken

Best to order from the à la carte menu |

TYPE OF FOOD	AVOID/LIMIT	BETTER CHOICES
Italian	Red sauces (usually high in potassium), white sauces (usually high in phosphorus)	Plain or meat-filled pasta (e.g., spaghetti, fettuccini, penne, tortellini, ravioli)
		Wine sauces like in chicken marsala
		Order sauce on the side
		Small portion (3 ounces) of clam and mussel sauces that are not tomato- or cream-based (better choices than red or white sauces)
		Salad, bread, very plain pasta, such as garlic and butter pasta
		One tablespoon of grated Parmesan cheese may be used for added flavor
Mediterranean	Spinach-filled phyllo pastries, sausage rolls and chiko rolls (very high in sodium), tabouleh, falafel, scalloped potatoes	Cream or white-wine sauces; grilled, pan-fried, or marinated meats, chicken, fish, or seafood; dishes served with rice; couscous; kebabs and skewered lean meats; risotto
Barbecue	Barbecue sauce, steak sauce, mustard, ketchup, horseradish, sausage, hot dogs, corn bread	Lean meat, chicken, fish, or seafood; French bread or garlic bread; grilled vegetables
		Marinades with wine, lemon juice, oil, vinegar, garlic, honey, herbs and spices
Entrées	Casseroles; sauces; gravies; heavily fried items; breaded or battered foods; cured or salted meats; omelets with cheese, ham, sausage, or bacon	Broiled or grilled lean meats and fish, omelets with vegetables, sandwiches with meat filling
Sides	Kale, spinach, potatoes or potato salad, tomatoes, mushrooms, winter squash, baked or fried beans, sauerkraut, vegetables in heavy creams or sauces	Peas, sweet peas, green beans, corn, cabbage, zucchini, eggplant, cauliflower, lentils; plain rice, jasmine rice, pastas, noodles
Dessert	Chocolate; nuts; coconut; cheesecake; custard; puddings; dried fruit, star fruit, cantaloupe, oranges; pies such as cream, minced, pumpkin, rhubarb, and pecan; ice cream	Low-potassium fresh fruit or canned fruit, sugar cookies, angel food cake, gelatin

Eating at Social Gatherings

Birthdays, weddings, graduations, picnics, and barbecues are wonderful occasions for getting together with family and friends. For people with kidney disease, these social gatherings can also mean tough choices about what to eat and drink. It is possible to enjoy them if you have a good plan in place and keep a positive attitude. Below are some kidney-healthy diet tips for social gatherings:

1. Don't go hungry.

Have a snack before you leave the house. Going to any event hungry will only set you up for disaster and will most likely lead to overeating. Having a high-protein snack beforehand—for example, half of a tuna fish sandwich—will make you feel a little full and help you make healthier choices.

2. Avoid high-sodium foods.

Salty foods will only make you thirsty, which will make you want to drink more than you probably should. Rather than choosing hot dogs or sausages, choose lower-sodium foods such as chicken and hamburgers. Go easy on the barbecue sauce and salad dressing, because they are very high in salt. If available, you can even ask for vegetables to be grilled.

3. Limit alcohol.

It is best to speak with your physician first about drinking alcohol. Alcoholic beverages also count toward your fluid intake.

4. Food safety is important.

Having kidney disease does put you at a higher risk for food-borne illnesses. Keep food at safe temperatures, wash produce well, and use separate cutting boards for raw and cooked meats.

5. Plan ahead.

Feel free to ask your family or friends about the menu. This way you can decide exactly what you want to eat. If it's not to your liking and doesn't fit with your diet, you can bring your own dish.

PART 2

KIDNEY-HEALTHY RECIPES

CHAPTER FIVE

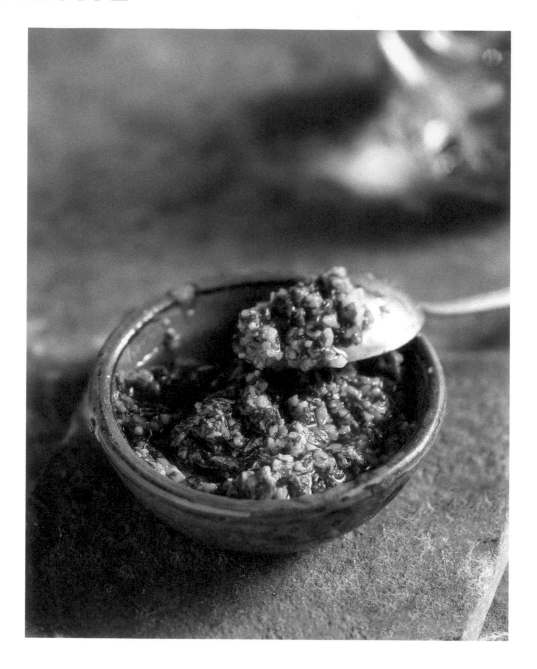

KITCHEN STAPLES

BALSAMIC VINAIGRETTE

Makes 3 cups [2 tablespoons = 1 serving] / Prep time: 5 minutes

Salads are a simple, healthy choice if you are watching your diet, so a delicious vinaigrette is a must-have. The herbs in this recipe can be switched out with your own favorites, but stick with fresh products whenever possible because dried herbs will not have as much flavor. The bright flecks of green from fresh herbs add an appealing bit of color to salad as well.

1½ cups extra virgin olive oil
1 cup good-quality balsamic vinegar
2 tablespoons chopped fresh parsley
2 tablespoons minced onion
1 teaspoon minced garlic
4 teaspoons chopped fresh basil
Freshly ground black pepper

1. In a large bowl, whisk together the olive oil and balsamic vinegar until the ingredients emulsify, about 1 minute.

2. Whisk in the parsley, onion, garlic, and basil.

3. Season with pepper.

4. Transfer the vinaigrette to a glass jar with a lid and store at room temperature for up to 2 weeks.

5. Shake before using.

PER SERVING Calories: 129; Fat: 14g; Carbohydrates: 2g; Phosphorus: 3mg; Potassium: 16mg; Sodium: 3mg; Protein: 0g

HOMEMADE MAYONNAISE

Makes 1 cup [1 tablespoon = 1 serving] / Prep time: 10 minutes

Mayonnaise is a traditional accompaniment for salads, burgers, and sandwiches. So a healthier version of the high-sodium, commercially prepared product is a handy addition to any kitchen. If you want to save a little time, whip up this recipe in a couple minutes with no whisking, using an immersion blender. Simply place your egg yolks, lemon juice, and mustard powder in a large jar that fits an immersion blender and blend for 15 seconds. Add the olive oil and blend for 15 seconds until the mayonnaise is thick and creamy.

2 egg yolks, at room temperature
1½ teaspoons freshly squeezed lemon juice
¼ teaspoon mustard powder
¾ cup olive oil

1. In a medium bowl, whisk together the yolks, lemon juice, and mustard for about 30 seconds or until well blended.

2. Add the olive oil in a thin, steady stream while whisking for about 3 minutes or until the oil is emulsified and the mayonnaise is thick.

3. Store the mayonnaise in the refrigerator in a sealed container for up to 1 week.

Ingredient tip: *Raw eggs are used in this recipe. It should not be served to pregnant women, young children, or anyone whose immune system is compromised. The best choice for the yolks in homemade mayonnaise is washed eggs from pasture-raised chickens. Most egg food poisoning cases have come from factory-farmed chickens, and there have been no cases reported in the United States from eggs laid by pasture-raised birds.*

PER SERVING Calories: 97; Fat: 11g; Carbohydrates: 0g; Phosphorus: 9mg; Potassium: 3mg; Sodium: 1mg; Protein: 0g

BALSAMIC REDUCTION

Makes ½ cup [1 tablespoon = 1 serving] / Cook time: 30 minutes

Balsamic vinegar has a rich, earthy flavor that is unmistakable and unique. This vinegar is crafted, rather than manufactured, from the pressings from grapes that are not used to make wine. The boiled-down pressings are aged under very stringent guidelines to produce balsamic vinegar. Although some balsamic vinegars are aged more than 100 years, you can use a younger, more inexpensive product for this reduction.

2 cups good-quality balsamic vinegar
1 tablespoon granulated sugar

1. Place a small saucepan over medium-high heat and whisk together the balsamic vinegar and sugar.
2. Bring the vinegar mixture to a boil.
3. Reduce the heat to low and simmer, stirring occasionally, for about 20 minutes or until the vinegar reduces.
4. Remove the vinegar reduction from the heat and allow it to cool completely.
5. Transfer the cooled reduction to a container and store at room temperature for up to 2 weeks.

Dialysis modification: *Balsamic reduction is meant to add an intense burst of flavor to meats, salads, and slices of grilled bread. To reduce the amount of potassium, you can use as little as 1 teaspoon and still enjoy the delicious, rich taste.*

PER SERVING Calories: 62; Fat: 0g; Carbohydrates: 12g; Phosphorus: 12mg; Potassium: 71mg; Sodium: 15mg; Protein: 0g

HERB PESTO

Makes 1½ cups [1 tablespoon = 1 serving] / Prep time: 10 minutes

Pesto can be created using a variety of base ingredients such as herbs, greens, and sun-dried tomatoes, as well as additions such as pine nuts, Parmesan cheese, and chile peppers, depending on the desired finished result. The herbs in this simple pesto are a guideline, so experiment with different choices and amounts until you get the taste you desire. Pesto is wonderful in soups and stews, as a topping for meats and poultry, or stirred into plain pasta for a simple and satisfying meal.

1 cup packed fresh basil leaves
½ cup packed fresh oregano leaves
½ cup packed fresh parsley leaves
2 garlic cloves
¼ cup olive oil
2 tablespoons freshly squeezed lemon juice

1. Put the basil, oregano, parsley, and garlic in a food processor and pulse for about 3 minutes or until very finely chopped.

2. Drizzle the olive oil into the pesto until a thick paste forms, scraping down the sides at least once.

3. Add the lemon juice and pulse until well blended.

4. Store the pesto in a sealed container in the refrigerator for up to 1 week.

PER SERVING Calories: 22; Fat: 2g; Carbohydrates: 0g; Phosphorus: 2mg; Potassium: 15mg; Sodium: 1mg; Protein: 0g

ALFREDO SAUCE

Serves 8 [¼ cup = 1 serving] / Prep time: 10 minutes / Cook time: 10 minutes

Creamy pasta sauces are typically an indulgence to be eaten on special occasions, with every forkful savored. This recipe tastes just as sinfully cheesy and creamy but without the hefty amounts of fat, calories, phosphorus, or sodium, so you can enjoy the sauce more often with family and friends. Wipe the bowl out with a chunk of crusty bread to soak up every last drop.

2 tablespoons unsalted butter
1½ tablespoons all-purpose flour
1 teaspoon minced garlic
1 cup plain unsweetened rice milk
¾ cup plain cream cheese
2 tablespoons Parmesan cheese
¼ teaspoon ground nutmeg
Freshly ground black pepper, for seasoning

1. In a medium saucepan over medium heat, melt the butter.
2. Whisk in the flour and garlic to form a paste, and continue whisking for 2 minutes to cook the flour.
3. Whisk in the rice milk and continue whisking for about 4 minutes or until the mixture is almost boiling and thick.
4. Whisk in the cream cheese, Parmesan cheese, and nutmeg for about 1 minute or until the sauce is smooth.
5. Remove the sauce from the heat and season with pepper.
6. Serve immediately over pasta.

PER SERVING Calories: 98; Fat: 7g; Carbohydrates: 6g; Phosphorus: 66mg; Potassium: 70mg; Sodium: 141mg; Protein: 3g

APPLE-CRANBERRY CHUTNEY

Makes 1 cup [1 tablespoon = 1 serving] / Prep time: 10 minutes / Cook time: 30 minutes

Chutneys sound old-fashioned and sweet, but most chutneys have complex flavors that range from mouth-scorching spicy to lip-puckering tart with only a hint of sweetness. This chutney is a milder variation that perfectly balances sweet and tart. You should keep a jar handy for chicken and pork recipes, as well as for a tasty snack on top of crackers.

1 large apple, peeled, cored, and sliced thin
½ cup granulated sugar
½ cup fresh cranberries
½ red onion, finely chopped
¼ cup apple juice
¼ cup apple cider vinegar
Freshly ground black pepper, for seasoning

1. In a medium saucepan over medium heat, stir together the apple, sugar, cranberries, onion, apple juice, and vinegar.

2. Bring the mixture to a boil, and then reduce the heat to low and cook, stirring frequently, for 25 to 30 minutes or until the cranberries are very tender.

3. Season with pepper.

4. Remove the chutney from the heat and chill in the refrigerator for about 3 hours or until completely cool.

5. Store the chutney in a sealed container in the refrigerator for up to 1 week.

PER SERVING Calories: 36; Fat: 0g; Carbohydrates: 9g; Phosphorus: 3mg; Potassium: 25mg; Sodium: 1mg; Protein: 0g

COOKED FOUR-PEPPER SALSA

Makes 4 cups [½ cup = 1 serving] / Prep time: 15 minutes / Cook time: 1 hour, 15 minutes

Red bell peppers are a popular choice if you are following a renal diet because they are low in potassium. This pretty-hued vegetable is also a nutritional powerhouse because it is an excellent source of vitamins A and C (both antioxidants), vitamin E, vitamin B$_6$, folate, and fiber. Red bell peppers also contain the antioxidants lycopene, and beta-cryptoxanthin, which offer protection against heart disease and lung cancer.

1 pound red bell peppers, boiled and chopped
2 small sweet banana peppers, chopped
1 small sweet onion, chopped
1 jalapeño pepper, finely chopped
1 green bell pepper, chopped
½ cup apple cider vinegar
2 teaspoons minced garlic
1 tablespoon granulated sugar
3 tablespoons chopped fresh cilantro

1. In a large saucepan, mix together the red bell peppers, banana peppers, onion, jalapeño pepper, green bell pepper, apple cider vinegar, garlic, and sugar over medium heat.

2. Bring the mixture to a boil, stirring frequently.

3. Reduce the heat to low and simmer for about 1 hour, stirring frequently.

4. Stir in the cilantro and simmer, stirring occasionally, for 15 minutes.

5. Remove the salsa from the heat and allow it to cool 15 to 20 minutes.

6. Transfer the salsa to a container and chill in the refrigerator until you are ready to use it, up to 1 week.

7. Serve cold with baked tortilla chips.

PER SERVING   Calories: 40; Fat: 0g; Carbohydrates: 8g; Phosphorus: 24mg; Potassium: 191mg; Sodium: 4mg; Protein: 1g

EASY CHICKEN STOCK

Makes 8 to 10 cups [1 cup = 1 serving] / Prep time: 15 minutes /
Cook time: 7 to 8 hours

Making chicken stock is an art that requires a large stockpot and patience. The ingredients that go into this staple are very flexible, so omit or add whatever you want as long as the carcass, water, and vinegar remain. The vinegar draws out important nutrients from the chicken bones that enhance the health benefits of making your own stock. If you use a raw carcass, roast the bones in the oven for a few hours to enhance the flavor before adding the carcass to your stockpot.

1 roasted chicken carcass, skin removed
Water
1 tablespoon apple cider vinegar
4 celery stalks, chopped into 2-inch pieces
2 sweet onions, peeled and quartered
2 carrots, cut into 2-inch chunks
2 garlic cloves, crushed
2 bay leaves
5 fresh thyme sprigs
5 fresh parsley stems
½ teaspoon black peppercorns

1. Put the chicken carcass in a large 4- to 6-quart stockpot, cutting it into smaller pieces to make it fit, if needed.
2. Cover the carcass with water until the liquid covers the carcass by about 1 inch, and add the apple cider vinegar.
3. Place the stockpot over medium heat until the liquid simmers and then reduce the heat to low so that it simmers very gently.
4. Simmer the carcass for 5 to 6 hours, adding more water if the top of the carcass gets exposed.
5. Skim off any accumulated foam on the stock. ▶

6. Add the celery, onion, carrots, garlic, bay leaves, thyme, parsley, and peppercorns to the stockpot.

7. Simmer for 2 hours, adding more water if required to keep the ingredients covered.

8. Strain the stock through a fine-mesh strainer and discard the solids.

9. Let the stock cool, and store in the refrigerator for up to 1 week or in the freezer for up to 6 months.

Dialysis modification: *When the stock is finished, add water to increase the volume and reduce the amount of potassium. As many as 3 or 4 cups of water will not dilute the chicken taste too much, but make sure to taste as you add water to reach an acceptable flavor.*

PER SERVING Calories: 38; Fat: 1g; Carbohydrates: 3g; Phosphorus: 72mg; Potassium: 197mg; Sodium: 72mg; Protein: 5g

CINNAMON APPLESAUCE

Makes 3 cups [½ cup = 1 serving] / Prep time: 10 minutes / Cook time: 30 minutes

Applesauce is a comfort food in a healthy package. The sweet, slightly tart, spiced goodness of this dish is perfect for a nutrition-packed snack, as breakfast, or even spooned over a simple grilled pork chop. Apples are full of fiber and rich in antioxidants. This recipe is even sweeter if you need to use up apples that are a wee bit past their prime.

8 apples, peeled, cored, and sliced thin
½ cup water
1 teaspoon ground cinnamon
¼ teaspoon ground nutmeg
Pinch ground allspice

1. Put the apples, water, cinnamon, nutmeg, and allspice in a medium saucepan over medium heat.

2. Heat the apple mixture, stirring frequently, for 25 to 30 minutes, or until the apples soften.

3. Remove the saucepan from the heat and use a potato masher to mash the apples to the desired texture.

4. Let the applesauce cool.

5. Store in the refrigerator for up to 1 week.

PER SERVING Calories: 106; Fat: 0g; Carbohydrates: 28g; Phosphorus: 24mg; Potassium: 196mg; Sodium: 0g; Protein: 1g

LEMON CURD

Makes 1½ cups [2 tablespoons = 1 serving] / Prep time: 15 minutes /
Cook time: 10 minutes

Lemon is one of the most popular taste profiles in the world, across many different cultures. This velvety curd has an intense lemon flavor accented by a touch of sweetness and rich butter. You can spread lemon curd on toast, fold it into whipped topping for a light dessert, or use it to top a bowl of fresh berries. Lemons are an excellent source of limonene, which has been shown to have antioxidant properties. Lemons also are an excellent source of vitamin C and folate.

6 large egg yolks
¾ cup granulated sugar
Zest of 4 lemons
Juice of 4 lemons
½ cup unsalted butter, cut into 1-inch pieces

1. Pour about 2 inches of water into a small saucepan and place over medium-high heat until the water simmers.

2. Reduce the heat to low so the water gently simmers, and place a medium stainless-steel bowl over the saucepan.

3. In the bowl, whisk together the egg yolks, sugar, lemon zest, and lemon juice for 8 to 10 minutes or until the mixture forms thick ribbons when you lift up the whisk.

4. Remove the bowl from the saucepan and whisk in the butter pieces, one at a time, until each is fully incorporated.

5. Pour the lemon curd through a fine-mesh strainer into another medium bowl. Use the back of a spoon to press through extra curd and squeeze out the zest.

6. Discard the zest in the strainer, and cover the lemon curd with plastic wrap that is pressed right onto the surface of the curd.

7. Chill in the refrigerator for about 3 hours or until set.

8. Store in the refrigerator in a sealed container for up to 1 week.

PER SERVING   Calories: 148; Fat: 10g; Carbohydrates: 14g; Phosphorus: 37mg; Potassium: 32mg; Sodium: 5g; Protein: 1g

TRADITIONAL BEEF STOCK

Makes 8 cups [1 cup = 1 serving] / Prep time: 15 minutes / Cook time: 13 hours

Most grocery stores have bones in their meat sections because bone broth and a back-to-basics attitude about diet has created a demand for this ingredient. You can also visit a butcher or a farmers' market to find good quality beef bones.

2 pounds beef bones (beef marrow, knuckle bones, or ribs)
1 celery stalk, chopped into 2-inch pieces
1 carrot, peeled and roughly chopped
½ sweet onion, peeled and quartered
3 garlic cloves, crushed
1 teaspoon black peppercorns
3 sprigs thyme
2 bay leaves
Water

1. Preheat the oven to 350°F.
2. Place the bones in a deep baking pan and roast them in the oven for 30 minutes, turning once.
3. Transfer the roasted bones to a large stockpot and add the celery, carrots, onion, garlic, peppercorns, thyme, bay leaves, and enough water to cover the bones by about 3 inches.
4. Reduce the heat to low and simmer the stock for at least 12 hours. Check the broth every hour for the first 4 hours to skim off any foam or impurities from the top.
5. Remove the pot from the heat and cool for 30 minutes.
6. Remove the large bones with tongs, and then strain the stock through a fine-mesh strainer and discard the solid bits in the strainer.
7. Pour the stock into jars or containers and allow it to cool completely.
8. Store the beef stock in sealed containers or jars in the refrigerator for up to 6 days, or in the freezer for up to 3 months.

PER SERVING Calories: 121; Fat: 5g; Carbohydrates: 2g; Phosphorus: 21mg; Potassium: 79mg; Sodium: 87mg; Protein: 4g

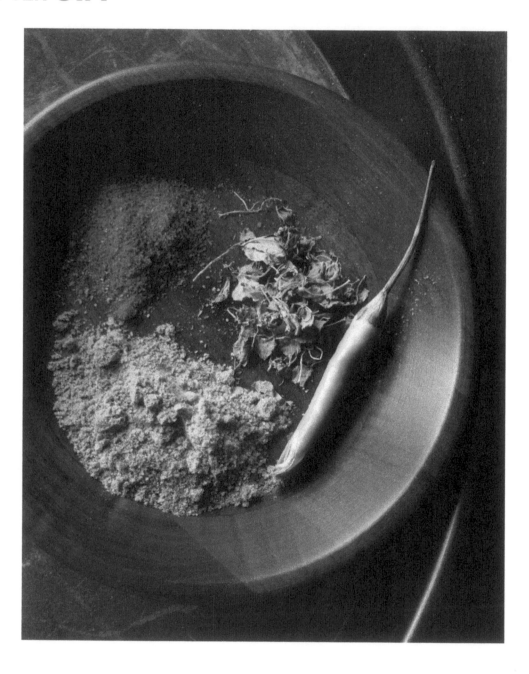

SPICE BLENDS AND SEASONINGS

FAJITA RUB

Makes ¼ cup [½ teaspoon = 1 serving] / Prep time: 5 minutes

Tex-Mex food is so popular it shows up in fine-dining restaurants across North America. Fajitas are one of the classic offerings in establishments featuring this cuisine. This combination of spices originated with Mexican workers in Texas in the 1930s, when they were given less-desirable cuts of beef such as flank or skirt steaks when steers were slaughtered. In Spanish, the word for girdle is faja, *which is the root of fajita.*

1½ teaspoons chili powder
1 teaspoon garlic powder
1 teaspoon roasted cumin seed
1 teaspoon dried oregano
½ teaspoon ground coriander
¼ teaspoon red pepper flakes

1. Put the chili powder, garlic powder, cumin seed, oregano, coriander, and red pepper flakes in a blender, and pulse until the ingredients are ground and well combined.

2. Transfer the spice mixture to a small container with a lid.

3. Store in a cool, dry place for up to 6 months.

PER SERVING Calories: 1; Fat: 0g; Carbohydrates: 0g; Phosphorus: 2mg; Potassium: 7mg; Sodium: 7mg; Protein: 0g

DRIED HERB RUB

Makes ⅓ cup [½ teaspoon = 1 serving] / Prep time: 5 minutes

The combination of herbs in this recipe can be changed according to your palate and depending on what you have in your pantry. Chicken, pork, and firm white fish are enhanced with a generous sprinkling of this mixture before grilling or baking. You can easily double the recipe if you find yourself using a lot of the rub.

1 tablespoon dried thyme

1 tablespoon dried oregano

1 tablespoon dried parsley

2 teaspoons dried basil

2 teaspoons ground coriander

2 teaspoons onion powder

1 teaspoon ground cumin

1 teaspoon garlic powder

1 teaspoon paprika

½ teaspoon cayenne pepper

1. Put the thyme, oregano, parsley, basil, coriander, onion powder, cumin, garlic powder, paprika, and cayenne pepper in a blender, and pulse until the ingredients are ground and well combined.

2. Transfer the rub to a small container with a lid.

3. Store in a cool, dry place for up to 6 months.

PER SERVING Calories: 3; Fat: 0g; Carbohydrates: 1g; Phosphorus: 3mg; Potassium: 16mg; Sodium: 1mg; Protein: 0g

MEDITERRANEAN SEASONING

Makes ⅓ cup [½ teaspoon = 1 serving] / Prep time: 5 minutes

This Mediterranean-inspired seasoning may conjure up images of sun-drenched patios, azure waters, and flavorful fresh food. Oregano is a popular herb in Greek cuisine and can be found growing in almost every kitchen garden in that country. Do not omit oregano from the seasoning mix if you want an authentic taste.

2 tablespoons dried oregano
1 tablespoon dried thyme
2 teaspoons dried rosemary, chopped finely or crushed
2 teaspoons dried basil
1 teaspoon dried marjoram
1 teaspoon dried parsley flakes

1. In a small bowl, mix together the oregano, thyme, rosemary, basil, marjoram, and parsley until well combined.
2. Transfer the seasoning mixture to a small container with a lid.
3. Store in a cool, dry place for up to 6 months.

PER SERVING Calories: 1; Fat: 0g; Carbohydrates: 0g; Phosphorus: 1mg; Potassium: 6mg; Sodium: 0mg; Protein: 0g

HOT CURRY POWDER

Makes 1¼ cups [1 tablespoon = 1 serving] / Prep time: 5 minutes

The yellowish-orange curry powder found in jars at the supermarket is a complex mix of many spices—not a single ingredient. A traditional South Asian curry contains turmeric, cumin, and coriander, with other spices thrown in depending on the region.

¼ cup ground cumin

¼ cup ground coriander

3 tablespoons turmeric

2 tablespoons sweet paprika

2 tablespoons ground mustard

1 tablespoon fennel powder

½ teaspoon green chili powder

2 teaspoons ground cardamom

1 teaspoon ground cinnamon

½ teaspoon ground cloves

1. Put the cumin, coriander, turmeric, paprika, mustard, fennel powder, green chili powder, cardamom, cinnamon, and cloves into a blender, and pulse until the ingredients are ground and well combined.

2. Transfer the curry powder to a small container with a lid.

3. Store in a cool, dry place for up to 6 months.

Dialysis modification: *Omit the sweet paprika to reduce the amount of potassium. It will change the color of the curry powder, but the other spices have a strong enough flavor to make up for the omission.*

PER SERVING Calories: 19; Fat: 1g; Carbohydrates: 3g; Phosphorus: 24mg; Potassium: 93mg; Sodium: 5mg; Protein: 1g

CAJUN SEASONING

Makes 1¼ cups [1 teaspoon = 1 serving] / Prep time: 5 minutes

Cajun cooking is native to Louisiana in the United States, but the original Cajuns were French people from Nova Scotia (Acadia) who were forced out of Canada by the British in 1755. A large group settled in south Louisiana and was eventually joined by more Cajuns looking for a safe haven. Cajun food is spicy, garlicky, and often features grilled meats or wild game.

½ cup sweet paprika

¼ cup garlic powder

3 tablespoons onion powder

3 tablespoons freshly ground black pepper

2 tablespoons dried oregano

1 tablespoon cayenne pepper

1 tablespoon dried thyme

1. Put the paprika, garlic powder, onion powder, black pepper, oregano, cayenne pepper, and thyme in a blender, and pulse until the ingredients are ground and well combined.

2. Transfer the seasoning mixture to a small container with a lid.

3. Store in a cool, dry place for up to 6 months.

PER SERVING Calories: 7; Fat: 0g; Carbohydrates: 2g; Phosphorus: 8mg; Potassium: 40mg; Sodium: 1mg; Protein: 0g

APPLE PIE SPICE

Makes ⅓ cup [1 teaspoon = 1 serving] / Prep time: 5 minutes

If you use pumpkin pie spice, this blend will taste and smell familiar. Pumpkins are not recommended on a renal diet, but apple pie can fill in. This spice mix can also be added to ½ cup of granulated sugar to create a delicious topping for hot buttered toast when you need a treat.

¼ cup ground cinnamon
2 teaspoons ground nutmeg
2 teaspoons ground ginger
1 teaspoon allspice
½ teaspoon ground cloves

1. In a small bowl, mix together the cinnamon, nutmeg, ginger, allspice, and cloves until the ingredients are well combined.

2. Transfer the spice mixture to a small container with a lid.

3. Store in a cool, dry place for up to 6 months.

PER SERVING Calories: 6; Fat: 0g; Carbohydrates: 1g; Phosphorus: 2mg; Potassium: 12mg; Sodium: 1mg; Protein: 0g

RAS EL HANOUT

Makes ½ cup [1 teaspoon = 1 serving] / Prep time: 5 minutes

Spices are a way of life in many North African regions, and the intoxicating scent of spice markets lingers in city streets. Many variations of ras el hanout spice mix exist. Some are tightly held secrets of families and restaurants in North Africa. Some variations include up to 100 different spices in the blend. This recipe is a simple version of the traditional mixture.

2 teaspoons ground nutmeg

2 teaspoons ground coriander

2 teaspoons ground cumin

2 teaspoons turmeric

2 teaspoons cinnamon

1 teaspoon cardamom

1 teaspoon sweet paprika

1 teaspoon ground mace

1 teaspoon freshly ground black pepper

1 teaspoon cayenne pepper

½ teaspoon ground allspice

½ teaspoon ground cloves

1. In a small bowl, mix together the nutmeg, coriander, cumin, turmeric, cinnamon, cardamom, paprika, mace, black pepper, cayenne pepper, allspice, and cloves until the ingredients are well combined.

2. Transfer the seasoning mixture to a small container with a lid.

3. Store in a cool, dry place for up to 6 months.

PER SERVING   Calories: 5; Fat: 0g; Carbohydrates: 1g; Phosphorus: 3mg; Potassium: 17mg; Sodium: 1mg; Protein: 0g

POULTRY SEASONING

Makes ½ cup [1 teaspoon = 1 serving] / Prep time: 5 minutes

Commercially prepared poultry seasonings are often very high in sodium because salt is thought to draw the juices out of the bird to produce a crackly, golden skin. Salt does draw the juices out of chicken and turkey, but you do not need it to create a lovely meal. Celery seed adds a salty flavor to this blend without the sodium.

2 tablespoons ground thyme

2 tablespoons ground marjoram

1 tablespoon ground sage

1 tablespoon ground celery seed

1 teaspoon ground rosemary

1 teaspoon freshly ground black pepper

1. In a small bowl, mix together the thyme, marjoram, sage, celery seed, rosemary, and pepper until the ingredients are well combined.

2. Transfer the seasoning mixture to a small container with a lid.

3. Store in a cool, dry place for up to 6 months.

PER SERVING Calories: 3; Fat: 0g; Carbohydrates: 0g; Phosphorus: 3mg; Potassium: 10mg; Sodium: 1mg; Protein: 0g

BERBERE SPICE MIX

Makes ½ cup [1 teaspoon = 1 serving] / Prep time: 5 minutes / Cook time: 5 minutes

This spice mix takes a little more work than just mixing ingredients in a bowl, but the result is worth all the effort. Berbere has its roots in Ethiopia, where its fiery taste is familiar even to children. Do not exclude the fenugreek seeds and dried chiles if you want to try an authentic-flavored blend.

1 tablespoon coriander seeds
1 teaspoon cumin seeds
1 teaspoon fenugreek seeds
¼ teaspoon black peppercorns
¼ teaspoon whole allspice berries
4 whole cloves
4 dried chiles, stemmed and seeded
¼ cup dried onion flakes
2 tablespoons ground cardamom
1 tablespoon sweet paprika
1 teaspoon ground ginger
½ teaspoon ground nutmeg
½ teaspoon ground cinnamon

1. In a small skillet over medium heat, add the coriander, cumin, fenugreek, peppercorns, allspice, and cloves.
2. Lightly toast the spices, swirling the skillet constantly, for about 4 minutes or until the spices are fragrant.
3. Remove the skillet from the heat and let the spices cool for about 10 minutes.
4. Transfer the toasted spices to a blender with the chiles and onion, and grind until the mixture is finely ground.
5. Transfer the ground spice mixture to a small bowl and stir together the cardamom, paprika, ginger, nutmeg, and cinnamon until thoroughly combined.
6. Store the spice mixture in a small container with a lid for up to 6 months.

PER SERVING Calories: 8; Fat: 0g; Carbohydrates: 2g; Phosphorus: 7mg; Potassium: 37mg; Sodium: 14mg; Protein: 0g

CREOLE SEASONING MIX

Makes ¼ cup [1 teaspoon = 1 serving] / Prep time: 5 minutes

Creole food is the urban equivalent of the more rural Cajun cuisine in Louisiana. Traditional Creole food uses tomatoes, which are not recommended on a renal diet, but you can still enjoy using this seasoning mix in recipes despite the tomato omission. Creole cuisine uses many high-quality ingredients made popular in upscale kitchens in New Orleans.

1 tablespoon sweet paprika

1 tablespoon garlic powder

2 teaspoons onion powder

2 teaspoons dried oregano

1 teaspoon cayenne pepper

1 teaspoon ground thyme

1 teaspoon freshly ground black pepper

1. In a small bowl, mix together the paprika, garlic powder, onion powder, oregano, cayenne pepper, thyme, and black pepper until the ingredients are well combined.

2. Transfer the seasoning mixture to a small container with a lid.

3. Store in a cool, dry place for up to 6 months.

PER SERVING Calories: 7; Fat: 0g; Carbohydrates: 2g; Phosphorus: 8mg; Potassium: 35mg; Sodium: 1mg; Protein: 0g

ADOBO SEASONING MIX

Makes 1¼ cups [1 teaspoon = 1 serving] / Prep time: 5 minutes

This mix varies depending on the region and is often used for meats and poultry, and as a marinade base for peppers or other vegetables. Dried citrus zest can be added to the mix for a Puerto Rican flair, or you can mix this blend with lemon juice or vinegar to create a wet rub for fish or pork.

4 tablespoons garlic powder

4 tablespoons onion powder

4 tablespoons ground cumin

3 tablespoons dried oregano

3 tablespoons freshly ground black pepper

2 tablespoons sweet paprika

2 tablespoons ground chili powder

1 tablespoon ground turmeric

1 tablespoon ground coriander

1. In a small bowl, mix together the garlic powder, onion powder, cumin, oregano, black pepper, paprika, chili powder, turmeric, and coriander until the ingredients are well combined.

2. Transfer the seasoning mixture to a small container with a lid and store in a cool, dry place for up to 6 months.

PER SERVING Calories: 8; Fat: 0g; Carbohydrates: 2g; Phosphorus: 9mg; Potassium: 38mg; Sodium: 12mg; Protein: 0g

HERBES DE PROVENCE

Makes 1 cup [1 teaspoon = 1 serving] / Prep time: 5 minutes

The banks of purple lavender stretching for miles in the French countryside are a breathtaking reminder that this fragrant flower is also delicious in food. You do not have to include lavender in this mix, but because it adds a unique flavor and can be purchased easily online, why leave it out? Make sure you purchase organic, culinary-grade lavender to avoid pesticide or chemical contamination.

½ cup dried thyme
3 tablespoons dried marjoram
3 tablespoons dried savory
2 tablespoons dried rosemary
2 teaspoons dried lavender flowers
1 teaspoon ground fennel

1. Put the thyme, marjoram, savory, rosemary, lavender, and fennel in a blender and pulse a few times to combine.

2. Transfer the herb mixture to a small container with a lid.

3. Store in a cool, dry place for up to 6 months.

PER SERVING Calories: 3; Fat: 0g; Carbohydrates: 1g; Phosphorus: 2mg; Potassium: 9mg; Sodium: 0mg; Protein: 0g

LAMB AND PORK SEASONING

Makes ½ cup [1 teaspoon = 1 serving] / Prep time: 5 minutes

Meats often need more assertive spicing than delicate fish or poultry, so seasoning with celery seed, onion, garlic, and lots of black pepper creates just the right taste. Bay leaves are often used whole in stews, soups, and sauces, but they can also be found ground in the spice section of most supermarkets.

¼ cup celery seed
2 tablespoons dried oregano
2 tablespoons onion powder
1 tablespoon dried thyme
1½ teaspoons garlic powder
1 teaspoon crushed bay leaf
1 teaspoon freshly ground black pepper
1 teaspoon ground allspice

1. Put the celery seed, oregano, onion powder, thyme, garlic powder, bay leaf, pepper, and allspice in a blender and pulse a few times to combine.

2. Transfer the herb mixture to a small container with a lid.

3. Store in a cool, dry place for up to 6 months.

PER SERVING Calories: 8; Fat: 0g; Carbohydrates: 1g; Phosphorus: 9mg; Potassium: 29mg; Sodium: 2mg; Protein: 0g

ASIAN SEASONING

Makes ½ cup [1 teaspoon = 1 serving] / Prep time: 5 minutes

Toasty-flavored sesame and exotic licorice-flavored anise combine with a mix of fragrant spices to create a seasoning blend that might become your new favorite. Seeds are not usually allowed if you are following a renal diet, but the quantity in this mix is tiny when divided into teaspoon-sized servings. You can omit the sesame seeds, but the loss in flavor will be significant.

2 tablespoons sesame seeds

2 tablespoons onion powder

2 tablespoons crushed star anise pods

2 tablespoons ground ginger

1 teaspoon ground allspice

½ teaspoon cardamom

½ teaspoon ground cloves

1. In a small bowl, mix together the sesame seeds, onion powder, star anise, ginger, allspice, cardamom, and cloves until well combined.

2. Transfer the spice mixture to a small container with a lid.

3. Store in a cool, dry place for up to 6 months.

PER SERVING Calories: 10; Fat: 0g; Carbohydrates: 1g; Phosphorus: 11mg; Potassium: 24mg; Sodium: 5mg; Protein: 0g

ONION SEASONING BLEND

Makes ½ cup [1 teaspoon = 1 serving] / Prep time: 5 minutes

Onion powder has an intense flavor without any of the bite that can be found in fresh onions. This seasoning blend has an unexpected sweet undertone, which is perfect for pork or sprinkling on roasted vegetables. You can also enjoy the taste of onions without the crying that can happen when cutting fresh alliums.

2 tablespoons onion powder
1 tablespoon dry mustard
2 teaspoons sweet paprika
2 teaspoons garlic powder
1 teaspoon dried thyme
½ teaspoon celery seeds
½ teaspoon freshly ground black pepper

1. In a small bowl, mix together the onion powder, mustard, paprika, garlic powder, thyme, celery seeds, and pepper until well combined.

2. Transfer the spice mixture to a small container with a lid.

3. Store in a cool, dry place for up to 6 months.

PER SERVING Calories: 5; Fat: 0g; Carbohydrates: 1g; Phosphorus: 6mg; Potassium: 17mg; Sodium: 1mg; Protein: 1g

COFFEE DRY RUB

Makes ¼ cup [1 teaspoon = 1 serving] / Prep time: 5 minutes

Coffee is typically something you enjoy in a mug in the morning, not an ingredient you rub on red meat. However, coffee adds a complexity to any flavoring mix and enhances the natural taste of beef. If you have a coffee grinder, grind your coffee right before mixing this rub together so the taste is intense.

1 tablespoon ground coffee

2 teaspoons ground cumin

2 teaspoons sweet paprika

2 teaspoons chili powder

1 teaspoon brown sugar

¼ teaspoon freshly ground black pepper

1. In a small bowl, mix together the coffee, cumin, paprika, chili powder, brown sugar, and pepper until well combined.

2. Transfer the rub to a small container with a lid.

3. Store in a cool, dry place for up to 6 months.

PER SERVING Calories: 5; Fat: 0g; Carbohydrates: 1g; Phosphorus: 5mg; Potassium: 32mg; Sodium: 18mg; Protein: 0g

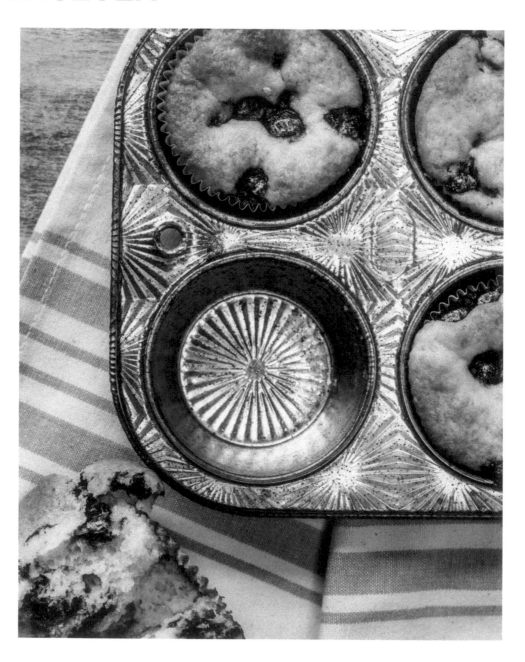

BREAKFAST

APPLE-CHAI SMOOTHIE

Serves 2 / Prep time: 5 minutes, plus 30 minutes to steep / Cook time: 5 minutes

Chai is redolent with warm spices such as ginger, cardamom, black peppercorns, fennel, cinnamon, and cloves. This tea is not only delicious but also a powerful antioxidant and may help support digestion. The taste of this smoothie is dependent on steeping the tea for at least 30 minutes.

1 cup unsweetened rice milk
1 chai tea bag
1 apple, peeled, cored, and chopped
2 cups ice

1. In a medium saucepan, heat the rice milk over low heat for about 5 minutes or until steaming.

2. Remove the milk from the heat and add the tea bag to steep.

3. Let the milk cool in the refrigerator with the tea bag for about 30 minutes and then remove tea bag, squeezing gently to release all the flavor.

4. Place the milk, apple, and ice in a blender and blend until smooth.

5. Pour into 2 glasses and serve.

PER SERVING   Calories: 88; Fat: 1g; Carbohydrates: 19g; Phosphorus: 74mg; Potassium: 92mg; Sodium: 47mg; Protein: 1g

BLUEBERRY-PINEAPPLE SMOOTHIE

Serves 2 / Prep time: 15 minutes

The sweetness in this smoothie comes from the pineapple, so if you enjoy a more tart breakfast drink, reduce the amount you use, or use slightly underripe fruit. If you are cutting up a fresh pineapple, remove the fibrous core before adding the fruit to your blender. Pineapple is an excellent source of vitamin C and a good source of dietary fiber, vitamin B_6, and copper.

1 cup frozen blueberries
½ cup pineapple chunks
½ cup English cucumber
½ apple
½ cup water

1. Put the blueberries, pineapple, cucumber, apple, and water in a blender and blend until thick and smooth.

2. Pour into 2 glasses and serve.

PER SERVING Calories: 87; Fat: 1g; Carbohydrates: 22g; Phosphorus: 28mg; Potassium: 192mg; Sodium: 3mg; Protein: 1g

WATERMELON-RASPBERRY SMOOTHIE

Serves 2 / Prep time: 10 minutes

The rosy pink color of this smoothie is delightful, and its breezy taste is a refreshing way to start your day. Try to keep the pale green inner rind of the watermelon when you cut it up for the smoothie, because 95 percent of its nutrition is found in that part of the melon. Watermelon is an excellent source of vitamins A and C and the antioxidants lycopene and beta-carotene.

½ cup boiled, cooled, and shredded red cabbage
1 cup diced watermelon
½ cup fresh raspberries
1 cup ice

1. Put the cabbage in a blender and pulse for 2 minutes or until it is finely chopped.
2. Add the watermelon and raspberries and pulse for about 1 minute or until very well combined.
3. Add the ice and blend until the smoothie is very thick and smooth.
4. Pour into 2 glasses and serve.

Dialysis modification: *The watermelon can be reduced by ½ cup to decrease the amount of potassium per serving by 50 mg.*

PER SERVING   Calories: 47; Fat: 0g; Carbohydrates: 11g; Phosphorus: 30mg; Potassium: 197mg; Sodium: 4mg; Protein: 1g

FESTIVE BERRY PARFAIT

Serves 4 / Prep time: 20 minutes, plus 1 hour to chill

Dust off your old sundae glasses, because these parfaits are spectacular when you see all the layers. Snowy cream cheese, crumbled golden cookies, and vibrant berries combine to create a breakfast for holiday weekends or even a festive dessert. The fruit layer can be anything from stewed rhubarb to peach slices or raspberries. You also can swap out the homemade meringue cookies with plain vanilla wafers.

1 cup vanilla rice milk, at room temperature
½ cup plain cream cheese, at room temperature
1 tablespoon granulated sugar
½ teaspoon ground cinnamon
1 cup crumbled Meringue Cookies (page 131)
2 cups fresh blueberries
1 cup sliced fresh strawberries

1. In a small bowl, whisk together the milk, cream cheese, sugar, and cinnamon until smooth.

2. Into 4 (6-ounce) glasses, spoon ¼ cup of crumbled cookie in the bottom of each.

3. Spoon ¼ cup of the cream cheese mixture on top of the cookies.

4. Top the cream cheese with ¼ cup of the berries.

5. Repeat in each cup with the cookies, cream cheese mixture, and berries.

6. Chill in the refrigerator for 1 hour and serve.

PER SERVING Calories: 243; Fat: 11g; Carbohydrates: 33g; Phosphorus: 84mg; Potassium: 189mg; Sodium: 145mg; Protein: 4g

MIXED-GRAIN HOT CEREAL

Serves 4 / Prep time: 10 minutes / Cook time: 25 minutes

The portion size of this hearty breakfast is quite small, but this cereal, combined with a piece of fruit, will keep you going from morning until lunch. Bulgur wheat is high in fiber, low in fat, and offers a nice nutty taste. Serve this cereal topped with syrup, unsalted butter, or a sprinkle of brown sugar.

2¼ cups water

1¼ cups vanilla rice milk

6 tablespoons uncooked bulgur

2 tablespoons uncooked whole buckwheat

1 cup peeled, sliced apple

6 tablespoons plain uncooked couscous

½ teaspoon ground cinnamon

1. In a medium saucepan over medium-high heat, heat the water and milk.

2. Bring to a boil, and add the bulgur, buckwheat, and apple.

3. Reduce the heat to low and simmer, stirring occasionally, for 20 to 25 minutes or until the bulgur is tender.

4. Remove the saucepan from the heat and stir in the couscous and cinnamon.

5. Let the saucepan stand, covered, for 10 minutes, then fluff the cereal with a fork before serving.

PER SERVING   Calories: 159; Fat: 1g; Carbohydrates: 34g; Phosphorus: 130mg; Potassium: 116mg; Sodium: 33mg; Protein: 4g

CORN PUDDING

Serves 6 / Prep time: 10 minutes / Cook time: 40 minutes

Corn is a staple food in the United States, and it has been used in every type of dish for centuries. Corn pudding is a classic recipe that has its roots in an English savory custard pudding brought over by settlers to New England. The Ener-G baking soda substitute in this recipe, which can be found online as well as in health food stores, does not contain the sodium, potassium, and phosphorus found in regular baking soda.

Unsalted butter, for greasing the baking dish

2 tablespoons all-purpose flour

½ teaspoon Ener-G baking soda substitute

3 eggs

¾ cup unsweetened rice milk, at room temperature

3 tablespoons unsalted butter, melted

2 tablespoons light sour cream

2 tablespoons granulated sugar

2 cups frozen corn kernels, thawed

1. Preheat the oven to 350°F.
2. Lightly grease an 8-by-8-inch baking dish with butter; set aside.
3. In a small bowl, stir together the flour and baking soda substitute; set aside.
4. In a medium bowl, whisk together the eggs, rice milk, butter, sour cream, and sugar.
5. Stir the flour mixture into the egg mixture until smooth.
6. Add the corn to the batter and stir until very well mixed.
7. Spoon the batter into the baking dish and bake for about 40 minutes or until the pudding is set.
8. Let the pudding cool for about 15 minutes and serve warm.

PER SERVING Calories: 175; Fat: 10g; Carbohydrates: 19g; Phosphorus: 111mg; Potassium: 170mg; Sodium: 62mg; Protein: 5g

RHUBARB BREAD PUDDING

Serves 6 / Prep time: 15 minutes, plus 30 minutes to soak / Cook time: 50 minutes

In medieval times, bread pudding was peasant food created to use up stale bread. Most dessert bread puddings are quite sweet, but this version is more tart, and would be lovely for a lazy weekend-morning breakfast. Rhubarb is used more like fruit in cooking, but it is actually a vegetable. It is an excellent source of fiber and vitamin C.

Unsalted butter, for greasing the baking dish
1½ cups unsweetened rice milk
3 eggs
½ cup granulated sugar
1 tablespoon cornstarch
1 vanilla bean, split
10 thick pieces white bread, cut into 1-inch chunks
2 cups chopped fresh rhubarb

1. Preheat the oven to 350°F.
2. Lightly grease an 8-by-8-inch baking dish with butter; set aside.
3. In a large bowl, whisk together the rice milk, eggs, sugar, and cornstarch.
4. Scrape the vanilla seeds into the milk mixture and whisk to blend.
5. Add the bread to the egg mixture and stir to completely coat the bread.
6. Add the chopped rhubarb and stir to combine.

7. Let the bread and egg mixture soak for 30 minutes.

8. Spoon the mixture into the prepared baking dish, cover with aluminum foil, and bake for 40 minutes.

9. Uncover the bread pudding and bake for an additional 10 minutes or until the pudding is golden brown and set.

10. Serve warm.

Dialysis modification: *Reduce the rhubarb to 1 cup to bring the potassium to less than 150 mg per serving. Or omit the rhubarb completely to bring the potassium to less than 75 mg per serving. The bread pudding is delicious without the rhubarb, but it will be less tart.*

PER SERVING   Calories: 197; Fat: 4g; Carbohydrates: 35g; Phosphorus: 109mg; Potassium: 192mg; Sodium: 159mg; Protein: 6g

CINNAMON-NUTMEG BLUEBERRY MUFFINS

Makes 12 muffins / Prep time: 15 minutes / Cook time: 30 minutes

Fresh blueberries are the best option for these muffins, because frozen berries can create an unfortunate purple-hued batter and add too much moisture. Blueberries are an excellent source of vitamin C and other antioxidants, and they are very high in fiber.

2 cups unsweetened rice milk

1 tablespoon apple cider vinegar

3½ cups all-purpose flour

1 cup granulated sugar

1 tablespoon Ener-G baking soda substitute

1 teaspoon ground cinnamon

½ teaspoon ground nutmeg

Pinch ground ginger

½ cup canola oil

2 tablespoons pure vanilla extract

2½ cups fresh blueberries

1. Preheat the oven to 375°F.
2. Line the cups of a muffin pan with paper liners; set aside.
3. In a small bowl, stir together the rice milk and vinegar; set aside for 10 minutes.
4. In a large bowl, stir together the flour, sugar, baking soda substitute, cinnamon, nutmeg, and ginger until well mixed. Add the oil and vanilla to the milk mixture and stir to blend.
5. Add the milk mixture to the dry ingredients and stir until just combined.
6. Fold in the blueberries. Spoon the muffin batter evenly into the cups.
7. Bake the muffins for 25 to 30 minutes or until golden and a toothpick inserted in the center of a muffin comes out clean.
8. Allow the muffins to cool for 15 minutes before serving.

PER SERVING Calories: 331; Fat: 11g; Carbohydrates: 52g; Phosphorus: 90mg; Potassium: 89mg; Sodium: 35mg; Protein: 6g

FRUIT AND CHEESE BREAKFAST WRAP

Serves 2 / Prep time: 10 minutes

If you need to get up and run out the door because of an activity-packed day, this tasty wrap is a perfect choice. If you don't have apples on hand, pears, strawberries, and peaches are also a delicious combination with the tart cheese. These wraps can be made the night before to save even more time.

2 (6-inch) flour tortillas
2 tablespoons plain cream cheese
1 apple, peeled, cored, and sliced thin
1 tablespoon honey

1. Lay both tortillas on a clean work surface and spread 1 tablespoon of cream cheese onto each tortilla, leaving about ½ inch around the edges.

2. Arrange the apple slices on the cream cheese, just off the center of the tortilla on the side closest to you, leaving about 1½ inches on each side and 2 inches on the bottom.

3. Drizzle the apples lightly with honey.

4. Fold the left and right edges of the tortillas into the center, laying the edge over the apples.

5. Taking the tortilla edge closest to you, fold it over the fruit and the side pieces. Roll the tortilla away from you, creating a snug wrap.

6. Repeat with the second tortilla.

PER SERVING Calories: 188; Fat: 6g; Carbohydrates: 33g; Phosphorus: 73mg; Potassium: 136mg; Sodium: 177mg; Protein: 4g

EGG-IN-THE-HOLE

Serves 2 / Prep time: 5 minutes / Cook time: 5 minutes

This simple breakfast takes about 5 minutes from fridge to plate and tastes incredibly rich and delicious. The egg white will spread under the butter-browned toasted bread, leaving a perfectly framed yolk. You can top this dish with the chopped herbs of your choice, but chives offer a nice flavor.

2 (½-inch-thick) slices Italian bread
¼ cup unsalted butter
2 eggs
2 tablespoons chopped fresh chives
Pinch cayenne pepper
Freshly ground black pepper

1. Using a cookie cutter or a small glass, cut a 2-inch round from the center of each piece of bread.

2. In a large nonstick skillet over medium-high heat, melt the butter.

3. Place the bread in the skillet, toast it for 1 minute, and then flip the bread over.

4. Crack the eggs into the holes the center of the bread and cook for about 2 minutes or until the eggs are set and the bread is golden brown.

5. Top with chopped chives, cayenne pepper, and black pepper.

6. Cook the bread for another 2 minutes.

7. Transfer an egg-in-the-hole to each plate to serve.

PER SERVING Calories: 304; Fat: 29g; Carbohydrates: 12g; Phosphorus: 119mg; Potassium: 109mg; Sodium: 204mg; Protein: 9g

SKILLET-BAKED PANCAKE

Serves 2 / Prep time: 15 minutes / Cook time: 20 minutes

If you are used to flat pancakes, the puffy appearance of this pancake might be a surprise when it comes out of the oven. Don't be alarmed if the pancake collapses before you cut it into servings—this is normal. Deflation of the pancake creates a creamy, pudding-like center. You can top this golden beauty with fruit, a drizzle of syrup, or a dollop of whipped topping.

2 eggs
½ cup unsweetened rice milk
½ cup all-purpose flour
¼ teaspoon ground cinnamon
Pinch ground nutmeg
Cooking spray, for greasing the skillet

1. Preheat the oven to 450°F.

2. In a medium bowl, whisk together the eggs and rice milk.

3. Stir in the flour, cinnamon, and nutmeg until blended but still slightly lumpy, but do not overmix.

4. Spray a 9-inch ovenproof skillet with cooking spray and place the skillet in the preheated oven for 5 minutes.

5. Remove the skillet carefully and pour the pancake batter into the skillet.

6. Return the skillet to the oven and bake the pancake for about 20 minutes or until it is puffed up and crispy on the edges.

7. Cut the pancake into halves to serve.

Dialysis modification: *If you need additional protein in this dish, whisk in an extra egg white. There will be no change in texture or taste.*

PER SERVING Calories: 161; Fat: 1g; Carbohydrates: 30g; Phosphorus: 73mg; Potassium: 106mg; Sodium: 79mg; Protein: 7g

STRAWBERRY–CREAM CHEESE STUFFED FRENCH TOAST

Serves 4 / Prep time: 20 minutes, plus overnight to soak / Cook time: 1 hour, 5 minutes

If you need something out of the ordinary to serve for breakfast or brunch, try this elegant creation. There is no mess or fuss in the morning because the entire recipe can be put together the night before and left to soak in the refrigerator. The next morning, simply pop the baking dish in the oven. In one hour, you can serve a golden, crispy, sweet treat to your family or guests.

Cooking spray, for greasing the baking dish
½ cup plain cream cheese
4 tablespoons strawberry jam
8 slices thick white bread
2 eggs, beaten
½ cup unsweetened rice milk
1 teaspoon pure vanilla extract
1 tablespoon granulated sugar
¼ teaspoon ground cinnamon

1. Spray an 8-by-8-inch baking dish with cooking spray; set aside.
2. In a small bowl, stir together the cream cheese and jam until well blended.
3. Spread 3 tablespoons of the cream cheese mixture onto 4 slices of bread and top with the remaining 4 slices to make sandwiches.
4. In a medium bowl, whisk together the eggs, milk, and vanilla until smooth.
5. Dip the sandwiches into the egg mixture and lay them in the baking dish.
6. Pour any remaining egg mixture over the sandwiches and sprinkle them evenly with sugar and cinnamon.
7. Cover the dish with foil and refrigerate overnight.

8. Preheat the oven to 350°F.

9. Bake the French toast, covered, for 1 hour.

10. Remove the foil and bake for 5 minutes more or until the French toast is golden.

11. Serve warm.

PER SERVING Calories: 233; Fat: 9g; Carbohydrates: 30g; Phosphorus: 102mg; Potassium: 104mg; Sodium: 270mg; Protein: 9g

SUMMER VEGETABLE OMELET

Serves 3 / Prep time: 15 minutes / Cook time: 10 minutes

A good-quality nonstick pan is crucial when making omelets, especially when working with only egg whites. This omelet incorporates one whole egg among the whites, so the omelet will set more easily. The vegetables in the dish can include whatever you have on hand, or you can chop up an assortment of fresh herbs instead.

4 egg whites

1 egg

2 tablespoons chopped fresh parsley

2 tablespoons water

Olive oil spray, for greasing the skillet

½ cup chopped and boiled red bell pepper

¼ cup chopped scallion, both green and white parts

Freshly ground black pepper

1. In a small bowl, whisk together the egg whites, egg, parsley, and water until well blended; set aside.

2. Generously spray a large nonstick skillet with olive oil spray, and place it over medium-high heat.

3. Sauté the peppers and scallion for about 3 minutes or until softened.

4. Pour the egg mixture into the skillet over the vegetables and cook, swirling the skillet, for about 2 minutes or until the edges of the egg start to set.

5. Lift up the set edges and tilt the pan so that the uncooked egg can flow underneath the cooked egg.

6. Continue lifting and cooking the egg for about 4 minutes or until the omelet is set.

7. Loosen the omelet with a spatula and fold it in half. Cut the folded omelet into 3 portions and transfer the omelets to serving plates.

8. Season with black pepper and serve.

PER SERVING   Calories: 77; Fat: 3g; Carbohydrates: 2g; Phosphorus: 67mg; Potassium: 194mg; Sodium: 229mg; Protein: 12g

CHEESY SCRAMBLED EGGS WITH FRESH HERBS

Serves 4 / Prep time: 15 minutes / Cook time: 10 minutes

Cream cheese, chopped fresh herbs, and tender chopped scallion elevate humble scrambled eggs to a new culinary level. The cheese will create luscious golden curds that make these eggs seem to melt in your mouth. You can add chopped, cooked chicken or vegetables such as asparagus and red bell pepper if you want a more substantial meal or need to feed more people. Serve on white toast.

3 eggs, at room temperature

2 egg whites, at room temperature

½ cup cream cheese, at room temperature

¼ cup unsweetened rice milk

1 tablespoon finely chopped scallion, green part only

1 tablespoon chopped fresh tarragon

2 tablespoons unsalted butter

Freshly ground black pepper

1. In a medium bowl, whisk together the eggs, egg whites, cream cheese, rice milk, scallions, and tarragon until well blended and smooth.

2. In a large skillet over medium-high heat, melt the butter, swirling to coat the skillet evenly.

3. Pour in the egg mixture and cook, stirring, for about 5 minutes or until the eggs are thick and the curds creamy. Season with pepper.

PER SERVING Calories: 221; Fat: 19g; Carbohydrates: 3g; Phosphorus: 119mg; Potassium: 140mg; Sodium: 193mg; Protein: 8g

EGG AND VEGGIE MUFFINS

Serves 4 / Prep time: 15 minutes / Cook time: 20 minutes

These muffins are more like mini crustless quiches, but they bake in muffin pans, so the name fits. You can double the recipe and make enough to freeze for quick, 2-minute microwavable meals later in the week. Egg muffins also can be wrapped in tortillas or stuffed in a pita with shredded lettuce for lunch or a filling snack.

Cooking spray, for greasing the muffin pans
4 eggs
2 tablespoons unsweetened rice milk
½ sweet onion, finely chopped
½ red bell pepper, finely chopped
1 tablespoon chopped fresh parsley
Pinch red pepper flakes
Pinch freshly ground black pepper

1. Preheat the oven to 350°F.

2. Spray 4 muffin pans with cooking spray; set aside.

3. In a large bowl, whisk together the eggs, milk, onion, red pepper, parsley, red pepper flakes, and black pepper until well combined.

4. Pour the egg mixture into the prepared muffin pans.

5. Bake 18 to 20 minutes or until the muffins are puffed and golden.

6. Serve warm or cold.

PER SERVING Calories: 84; Fat: 5g; Carbohydrates: 3g; Phosphorus: 110mg; Potassium: 117mg; Sodium: 75mg; Protein: 7g

CURRIED EGG PITA POCKETS

Serves 4/ Prep time: 15 minutes / Cook time: 5 minutes

Pitas are handy, portable containers for an assortment of nutritious fillings. Make sure you purchase pita bread that is designed to open up (e.g., Greek-style pitas) because some pitas do not separate easily and are used more as a wrap or flatbread.

3 eggs, beaten

1 scallion, both green and white parts, finely chopped

½ red bell pepper, finely chopped

2 teaspoons unsalted butter

1 teaspoon curry powder

½ teaspoon ground ginger

2 tablespoons light sour cream

2 (4-inch) plain pita bread pockets, halved

½ cup julienned English cucumber

1 cup roughly chopped watercress

1. In a small bowl, whisk together the eggs, scallion, and red pepper until well blended.

2. In a large nonstick skillet over medium heat, melt the butter.

3. Pour the egg mixture into the skillet and cook for about 3 minutes or until the eggs are just set, swirling the skillet but not stirring. Remove the eggs from the heat; set aside.

4. In a small bowl, stir together the curry powder, ginger, and sour cream until well blended.

5. Evenly divide the curry sauce among the 4 halves of the pita bread, spreading it out on one inside edge.

6. Divide the cucumber and watercress evenly between the halves.

7. Spoon the eggs into the halves, dividing the mixture evenly, to serve.

PER SERVING Calories: 127; Fat: 7g; Carbohydrates: 10g; Phosphorus: 108mg; Potassium: 169mg; Sodium: 139mg; Protein: 7g

CHAPTER EIGHT

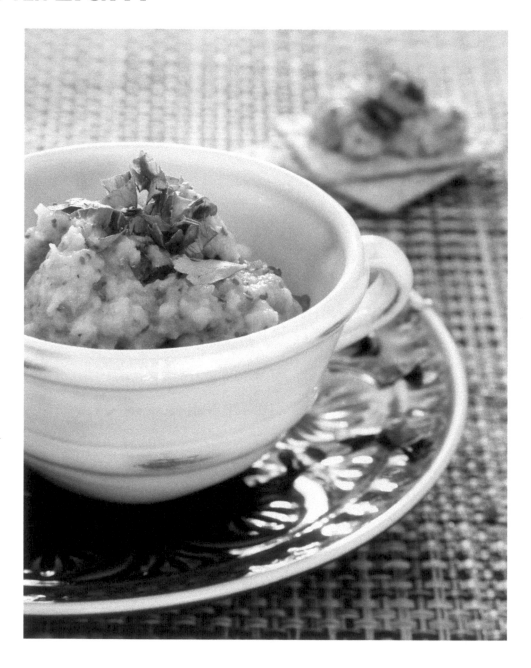

SNACKS

ROASTED ONION GARLIC DIP

Serves 6 [¼ cup = 1 serving] / Prep time: 15 minutes, plus 1 hour to chill /
Cook time: 1 hour

Roasting vegetables removes any bitterness, leaving only a rich, sweet flavor that is fabulous in recipes such as this robust, versatile dip. If the garlic cloves are very young and green, boil them in milk first for 5 minutes, rinse them, and then drizzle the cloves with oil. This process will draw out some of the overwhelmingly sharp garlic taste before roasting. Serve this dip with vegetables or pita triangles.

1 large sweet onion, peeled and cut into eighths
8 garlic cloves
2 teaspoons olive oil
½ cup light sour cream
1 tablespoon fresh lemon juice
1 tablespoon chopped fresh parsley
1 teaspoon chopped fresh thyme
Freshly ground black pepper

1. Preheat the oven to 425°F.
2. In a small bowl, toss the onion and garlic with the olive oil.
3. Transfer the onion and garlic to a piece of aluminum foil and wrap the vegetables loosely in a packet.
4. Place the foil packet on a small baking sheet and place the sheet in the oven.
5. Roast the vegetables for 50 minutes to 1 hour, or until they are very fragrant and golden.

6. Remove the packet from the oven and allow it to cool for 15 minutes.

7. In a medium bowl, stir together the sour cream, lemon juice, parsley, thyme, and black pepper.

8. Open the foil packet carefully and transfer the vegetables to a cutting board.

9. Chop the vegetables and add them to the sour cream mixture. Stir to combine.

10. Cover the dip and chill in the refrigerator for 1 hour before serving.

PER SERVING Calories: 44; Fat: 3g; Carbohydrates: 5g; Phosphorus: 22mg; Potassium: 79mg; Sodium: 10mg; Protein: 1g

BABA GHANOUSH

Serves 6 / Prep time: 20 minutes / Cook time: 30 minutes

Baba ghanoush is a dip that is similar to hummus, but eggplant is the star attraction. Eggplant can get very oily when it is cooked because it soaks up fat like a sponge, so make sure to brush it lightly with oil. You also can make a double batch of this recipe and use a couple of spoonfuls as an easy pasta sauce.

1 medium eggplant, halved and scored with a crosshatch pattern on the cut sides
1 tablespoon olive oil, plus extra for brushing
1 large sweet onion, peeled and diced
2 garlic cloves, halved
1 teaspoon ground cumin
1 teaspoon ground coriander
1 tablespoon lemon juice
Freshly ground black pepper

1. Preheat the oven to 400°F.
2. Line 2 baking sheets with parchment paper.
3. Brush the eggplant halves with olive oil and place them, cut-side down, on 1 baking sheet.
4. In a small bowl, mix together the onion, garlic, 1 tablespoon olive oil, cumin, and coriander.
5. Spread the seasoned onions on the other baking sheet.
6. Place both baking sheets in the oven and roast the onions for about 20 minutes and the eggplant for 30 minutes, or until softened and browned.
7. Remove the vegetables from the oven and scrape the eggplant flesh into a bowl.
8. Transfer the onions and garlic to a cutting board and chop coarsely; add to the eggplant.
9. Stir in the lemon juice and pepper.
10. Serve warm or chilled.

PER SERVING Calories: 45; Fat: 2g; Carbohydrates: 6g; Phosphorus: 23mg; Potassium: 195mg; Sodium: 3mg; Protein: 1g

CHEESE-HERB DIP

Serves 8 [3 tablespoons = 1 serving] / Prep time: 20 minutes

An easy, never-fails-to-please dip is a valuable addition to your culinary toolbox. If you are attending a neighborhood block party, having guests over for a family event, or you want something delicious on hand for movie night at home, this dip is a perfect choice. A bit of finely chopped vegetables or jalapeño peppers would also work with the base ingredients, so feel free to experiment with the recipe. Serve with cut vegetables.

1 cup cream cheese

½ cup unsweetened rice milk

½ scallion, green part only, finely chopped

1 tablespoon chopped fresh parsley

1 tablespoon chopped fresh basil

1 tablespoon freshly squeezed lemon juice

1 teaspoon minced garlic

½ teaspoon chopped fresh thyme

¼ teaspoon freshly ground black pepper

1. In a medium bowl, mix together the cream cheese, milk, scallion, parsley, basil, lemon juice, garlic, thyme, and pepper until well combined.

2. Store the dip in a sealed container in the refrigerator for up to 1 week.

PER SERVING Calories: 108; Fat: 10g; Carbohydrates: 3g; Phosphorus: 40mg; Potassium: 52mg; Sodium: 112mg; Protein: 2g

SPICY KALE CHIPS

Serves 6 / Prep time: 20 minutes / Cook time: 25 minutes

Kale has become a phenomenon in the last few decades, going from a food eaten only by health fanatics to a mainstream grocery item consumed by just about everyone. Kale chips are surprisingly crunchy, richly flavored, and are best eaten immediately if you are making your own. The trick to crispy chips is to very thoroughly dry the kale leaves and make sure the oil is massaged evenly into every leaf before baking.

2 cups kale
2 teaspoons olive oil
¼ teaspoon chili powder
Pinch cayenne pepper

1. Preheat the oven to 300°F.
2. Line 2 baking sheets with parchment paper; set aside.
3. Remove the stems from the kale and tear the leaves into 2-inch pieces.
4. Wash the kale and dry it completely.
5. Transfer the kale to a large bowl and drizzle with olive oil.
6. Use your hands to toss the kale with the oil, taking care to coat each leaf evenly.
7. Season the kale with chili powder and cayenne pepper and toss to combine thoroughly.
8. Spread the seasoned kale in a single layer on each baking sheet. Do not overlap the leaves.
9. Bake the kale, rotating the pans once, for 20 to 25 minutes or until it is crisp and dry.
10. Remove the trays from the oven and allow the chips to cool on the trays for 5 minutes.
11. Serve immediately.

PER SERVING Calories: 24; Fat: 2g; Carbohydrates: 2g; Phosphorus: 21mg; Potassium: 111mg; Sodium: 13g; Protein: 1g

CINNAMON TORTILLA CHIPS

Serves 6 / Prep time: 15 minutes / Cook time: 10 minutes

Cinnamon adds spice to savory and sweet dishes in a variety of different cuisines. Ground cinnamon comes from the bark of the cinnamon tree. Cinnamon may play a role in treating and healing chronic wounds because of the essential oils found in the bark. It also may help improve blood sugar and cholesterol levels in people with type 2 diabetes.

2 teaspoons granulated sugar
½ teaspoon ground cinnamon
Pinch ground nutmeg
3 (6-inch) flour tortillas
Cooking spray, for coating the tortillas

1. Preheat the oven to 350°F.
2. Line a baking sheet with parchment paper.
3. In a small bowl, stir together the sugar, cinnamon, and nutmeg.
4. Lay the tortillas on a clean work surface and spray both sides of each lightly with cooking spray.
5. Sprinkle the cinnamon sugar evenly over both sides of each tortilla.
6. Cut the tortillas into 16 wedges each and place them on the baking sheet.
7. Bake the tortilla wedges, turning once, for about 10 minutes or until crisp.
8. Cool the chips and store in a sealed container at room temperature for up to 1 week.

PER SERVING Calories: 51; Fat: 1g; Carbohydrates: 9g; Phosphorus: 29mg; Potassium: 24mg; Sodium: 103mg; Protein: 1g

SWEET AND SPICY KETTLE CORN

Serves 8 / Prep time: 1 minute / Cook time: 5 minutes

Microwave popcorn is an incredibly popular snack, but its ingredients and cooking process have caused concern in recent years. This recipe uses an old-fashioned stove-top technique that allows you to add the ingredients and flavorings you want. Take care not to allow the pot to get too hot, or the sugar will burn instead of caramelize.

3 tablespoons olive oil
1 cup popcorn kernels
½ cup brown sugar
Pinch cayenne pepper

1. Place a large pot with lid over medium heat and add the olive oil with a few popcorn kernels.

2. Shake the pot lightly until the popcorn kernels pop. Add the rest of the kernels and sugar to the pot.

3. Pop the kernels with the lid on the pot, shaking constantly, until they are all popped.

4. Remove the pot from the heat and transfer the popcorn to a large bowl.

5. Toss the popcorn with the cayenne pepper and serve.

PER SERVING Calories: 186; Fat: 6g; Carbohydrates: 30g; Phosphorus: 85mg; Potassium: 90mg; Sodium: 5mg; Protein: 3g

BLUEBERRIES AND CREAM ICE POPS

Makes 6 pops / Prep time: 10 minutes, plus 3 hours to freeze

Ice pops are a cheerful treat. They evoke memories of sunny childhood summers spent licking ice pops that dripped down your hand and onto scuffed sneakers. These homemade ice pops are not packed with sugar, dyes, and preservatives. You can use any type of fruit, such as strawberries, raspberries, peaches, and watermelon, for the base.

3 cups fresh blueberries
1 teaspoon freshly squeezed lemon juice
¼ cup unsweetened rice milk
¼ cup light sour cream
¼ cup granulated sugar
½ teaspoon pure vanilla extract
¼ teaspoon ground cinnamon

1. Put the blueberries, lemon juice, rice milk, sour cream, sugar, vanilla, and cinnamon in a blender and purée until smooth.
2. Spoon the mixture into ice-pop molds and freeze for 3 to 4 hours or until very firm.

PER SERVING   Calories: 78; Fat: 1g; Carbohydrates: 18g; Phosphorus: 20mg; Potassium: 55mg; Sodium: 12mg; Protein: 1g

CANDIED GINGER ICE MILK

Makes 4 cups / Prep time: 20 minutes, plus 1 hour to freeze / Cook time: 15 minutes

Ice milk is a refreshing version of ice cream, and you will only need a small portion of this cool treat to satisfy your taste buds. If you do not have an ice-cream maker, pour the mixture in a metal baking pan and place it in the freezer. Stir, and then scrape, the liquid as it freezes, creating an ice cream–like texture.

4 cups vanilla rice milk

½ cup granulated sugar

1 (4-inch) piece fresh ginger, peeled and sliced thin

¼ teaspoon ground nutmeg

¼ cup finely chopped candied ginger

1. In a large saucepan over medium heat, stir together the milk, sugar, and fresh ginger.

2. Heat the milk mixture, stirring occasionally, for about 5 minutes or until it is almost boiling.

3. Turn down the heat to low and simmer for 15 minutes.

4. Remove the milk mixture from the heat and add the ground nutmeg. Let the mixture sit for 1 hour to infuse the flavor.

5. Strain the milk mixture through a fine sieve into a medium bowl to remove the ginger.

6. Add the candied ginger, and place the mixture in the refrigerator to chill completely.

7. Freeze the ginger ice in an ice-cream maker according to the manufacturer's instructions.

8. Store the finished treat in the freezer in a sealed container for up to 3 months.

PER SERVING Calories: 108; Fat: 1g; Carbohydrates: 24g; Phosphorus: 68mg; Potassium: 45mg; Sodium: 47mg; Protein: 0g

MERINGUE COOKIES

Makes 24 cookies / Prep time: 30 minutes / Cook time: 30 minutes

Meringue cookies have a history that stretches back centuries. They appear in a French document from 1604, as well as in antique cookbooks in other countries. This recipe is a basic French meringue that does not require the candy thermometer or bain-marie needed in the Italian and Swiss versions. Make sure your egg whites are completely yolk-free or they will not whip up to the right texture and height. Also, your whisk or beaters need to be completely free of fat.

4 egg whites, at room temperature
1 cup granulated sugar
1 teaspoon pure vanilla extract
1 teaspoon almond extract

1. Preheat the oven to 300°F.
2. Line 2 baking sheets with parchment; set aside.
3. In a large stainless steel bowl, beat the egg whites until stiff peaks form.
4. Add the granulated sugar 1 tablespoon at a time, beating well to incorporate after each addition, until all the sugar is used and the meringue is thick and glossy.
5. Beat in the vanilla extract and almond extract.
6. Using a tablespoon, drop the meringue batter onto the baking sheets, spacing the cookies evenly.
7. Bake the cookies for about 30 minutes or until they are crisp.
8. Remove the cookies from the oven and let them cool on wire racks.
9. Store the cookies in an airtight container at room temperature for up to 1 week.

PER SERVING Calories: 36; Fat: 0g; Carbohydrates: 8g; Phosphorus: 1mg; Potassium: 10mg; Sodium: 9mg; Protein: 1g

CORN BREAD

Serves 10 / Prep time: 10 minutes / Cook time: 20 minutes

Corn bread is sometimes thought to be unhealthy because many chefs and home cooks add fat- and sodium-laden ingredients such as bacon and heaps of cheese. This recipe has all the buttery, sweet flavor of traditional corn bread without the unhealthy additions. You can add chopped jalapeño pepper or bits of roasted red bell pepper for a different, more complex taste.

Cooking spray, for greasing the baking dish
1¼ cups yellow cornmeal
¾ cup all-purpose flour
1 tablespoon Ener-G baking soda substitute
½ cup granulated sugar
2 eggs
1 cup unsweetened, unfortified rice milk
2 tablespoons olive oil

1. Preheat the oven to 425°F.

2. Lightly spray an 8-by-8-inch baking dish with cooking spray; set aside.

3. In a medium bowl, stir together the cornmeal, flour, baking soda substitute, and sugar.

4. In a small bowl, whisk together the eggs, rice milk, and olive oil until blended.

5. Add the wet ingredients to the dry ingredients and stir until well combined.

6. Pour the batter into the baking dish and bake for about 20 minutes or until golden and cooked through.

7. Serve warm.

PER SERVING   Calories: 198; Fat: 5g; Carbohydrates: 34g; Phosphorus: 88mg; Potassium: 94mg; Sodium: 25mg; Protein: 4g

ROASTED RED PEPPER AND CHICKEN CROSTINI

Serves 4 / Prep time: 10 minutes / Cook time: 5 minutes

Crostini and bruschetta are similar, but bruschetta usually has vegetable- or fruit-based toppings and crostini can be also topped with meats, fish, or poultry. The best crostini are made with bread that has been brushed with olive oil and grilled, so if you want to fire up your barbecue to create this recipe, the results will be spectacular. Make sure you grill both sides for the perfect crunch.

2 tablespoons olive oil
½ teaspoon minced garlic
4 slices French bread
1 roasted red bell pepper, chopped
4 ounces cooked chicken breast, shredded
½ cup chopped fresh basil

1. Preheat the oven to 400°F.

2. Line a baking sheet with aluminum foil.

3. In a small bowl, mix together the olive oil and garlic.

4. Brush both sides of each piece of bread with the olive oil mixture.

5. Place the bread on the baking sheet and toast in the oven, turning once, for about 5 minutes or until both sides are golden and crisp.

6. In a medium bowl, stir together the red pepper, chicken, and basil.

7. Top each toasted bread slice with the red pepper mixture and serve.

PER SERVING Calories: 184; Fat: 8g; Carbohydrates: 19g; Phosphorus: 87mg; Potassium: 152mg; Sodium: 175mg; Protein: 9g

CUCUMBER-WRAPPED VEGETABLE ROLLS

Serves 8 / Prep time: 30 minutes

Creating the perfect vegetable-wrapped roll hinges on the correct thinness of the vegetable you use as a wrapper. Cutting thin cucumber strips is much easier if you use a peeler, cheese cutter, or mandoline. A mandoline is a kitchen tool that slices very thin strips, makes batons, and cuts a pretty crosshatch using parallel and perpendicular blades. If you prepare a lot of fruits or vegetables, a mandoline is a smart investment.

½ cup finely shredded red cabbage

½ cup grated carrot

¼ cup julienned red bell pepper

¼ cup julienned scallion, both green and white parts

¼ cup chopped cilantro

1 tablespoon olive oil

¼ teaspoon ground cumin

¼ teaspoon freshly ground black pepper

1 English cucumber, sliced into 8 very thin strips with a vegetable peeler

1. In a medium bowl, toss together the cabbage, carrot, red pepper, scallion, cilantro, olive oil, cumin, and black pepper until well mixed.

2. Evenly divide the vegetable filling among the cucumber strips, placing the filling close to one end of the strip.

3. Roll up the cucumber strips around the filling and secure with a wooden pick.

4. Repeat with each cucumber strip.

PER SERVING Calories: 26; Fat: 2g; Carbohydrates: 3g; Phosphorus: 14mg; Potassium: 95mg; Sodium: 7mg; Protein: 0g

ANTOJITOS

Serves 8 / Prep time: 20 minutes

Antojitos, loosely translated, means "little cravings," which is accurate because these tempting spirals are addictive. The ingredients vary regionally, highlighting local cheeses, meats, and vegetables. These snacks are also called botanas in the Yucatán Peninsula. Although often served cold, you can pop the cut spirals under the broiler to melt the cheese.

6 ounces plain cream cheese, at room temperature

½ jalapeño pepper, finely chopped

½ scallion, green part only, chopped

¼ cup finely chopped red bell pepper

½ teaspoon ground cumin

½ teaspoon ground coriander

½ teaspoon chili powder

3 (8-inch) flour tortillas

1. In a medium bowl, mix together the cream cheese, jalapeño pepper, scallion, red bell pepper, cumin, coriander, and chili powder until well blended.

2. Divide the cream cheese mixture evenly among the 3 tortillas, spreading the cheese in a thin layer and leaving a ¼-inch edge all the way around.

3. Roll the tortillas like a jelly roll and wrap each tightly in plastic wrap.

4. Refrigerate the rolls for about 1 hour or until they are set.

5. Cut the tortilla rolls into 1-inch pieces and arrange them on a plate to serve.

PER SERVING Calories: 110; Fat: 8g; Carbohydrates: 7g; Phosphorus: 47mg; Potassium: 72mg; Sodium: 215mg; Protein: 2g

CHICKEN-VEGETABLE KEBABS

Serves 4 / Prep time: 15 minutes, plus 1 hour to marinate / Cook time: 12 minutes

These colorful kebabs are not meant to be anything more than a snack, so if you want to eat them as a meal, have two each instead of one. The onion can be tricky to get on the skewer as wedges, so you may want to use pearl onions instead. These little onions will fit perfectly on the skewer without separating into layers.

2 tablespoons olive oil
2 tablespoons freshly squeezed lemon juice
½ teaspoon minced garlic
½ teaspoon chopped fresh thyme
4 ounces boneless, skinless chicken breast, cut into 8 pieces
1 small summer squash, cut into 8 pieces
½ medium onion, cut into 8 pieces

1. In a medium bowl, stir together the olive oil, lemon juice, garlic, and thyme.

2. Add the chicken to the bowl and stir to coat.

3. Cover the bowl with plastic wrap and place the chicken in the refrigerator to marinate for 1 hour.

4. Thread the squash, onion, and chicken pieces onto 4 large skewers, evenly dividing the vegetables and meat among the skewers.

5. Heat a barbecue to medium and grill the skewers, turning at least 2 times, for 10 to 12 minutes or until the chicken is cooked through.

PER SERVING Calories: 106; Fat: 8g; Carbohydrates: 3g; Phosphorus: 77mg; Potassium: 199mg; Sodium: 14mg; Protein: 7g

FIVE-SPICE CHICKEN LETTUCE WRAPS

Serves 8 / Prep time: 30 minutes

Lettuce wraps are a common street food in Asia, filled with exotic ingredients and spices. Boston lettuce leaves are the best choice for the wrap part of the recipe because they are thin and do not have a stiff rib down the center. Green or red-leaf lettuce also works well if you use the outer leaves.

6 ounces cooked chicken breast, minced

1 scallion, both green and white parts, chopped

½ red apple, cored and chopped

½ cup bean sprouts

¼ English cucumber, finely chopped

Juice of 1 lime

Zest of 1 lime

2 tablespoons chopped fresh cilantro

½ teaspoon Chinese five-spice powder

8 Boston lettuce leaves

1. In a large bowl, mix together the chicken, scallions, apple, bean sprouts, cucumber, lime juice, lime zest, cilantro, and five-spice powder.

2. Spoon the chicken mixture evenly among the 8 lettuce leaves.

3. Wrap the lettuce around the chicken mixture and serve.

PER SERVING Calories: 51; Fat: 2g; Carbohydrates: 2g; Phosphorus: 56mg; Potassium: 110mg; Sodium: 16mg; Protein: 7g

CHAPTER NINE

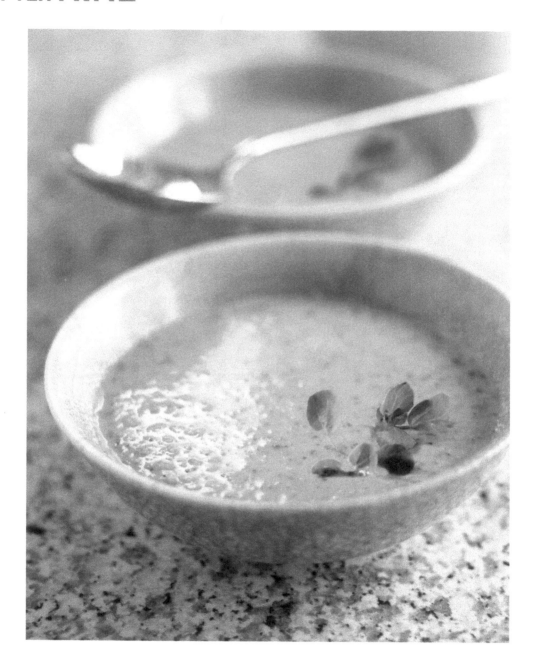

SOUPS AND STEWS

FRENCH ONION SOUP

Serves 4 / Prep time: 20 minutes / Cook time: 50 minutes

Creating a perfect French onion soup is a matter of pride for professional chefs, and the proper technique is the topic of heated arguments. The need to caramelize the onions is the only point that is agreed upon by most chefs, so try to devote adequate time to that step in this recipe. If your onions are very young and full of liquid, caramelization might need to be helped along by a tablespoon of granulated sugar.

2 tablespoons unsalted butter
4 Vidalia onions, sliced thin
2 cups Easy Chicken Stock (page 77)
2 cups water
1 tablespoon chopped fresh thyme
Freshly ground black pepper

1. In a large saucepan over medium heat, melt the butter.
2. Add the onions to the saucepan and cook them slowly, stirring frequently, for about 30 minutes or until the onions are caramelized and tender.
3. Add the chicken stock and water, and bring the soup to a boil.
4. Reduce the heat to low and simmer the soup for 15 minutes.
5. Stir in the thyme and season the soup with pepper.
6. Serve piping hot.

PER SERVING Calories: 90; Fat: 6g; Carbohydrates: 7g; Phosphorus: 22mg; Potassium: 192mg; Sodium: 57mg; Protein: 2g

CREAM OF WATERCRESS SOUP

Serves 4 / Prep time: 15 minutes / Cook time: 1 hour, 10 minutes

The gorgeous pastel color of this elegant soup and the lush accent flavor of roasted garlic make this dish a perfect recipe for company. You can certainly make it for a simple family meal, but set the table with fine china and heavy silverware to do the soup justice.

6 garlic cloves
½ teaspoon olive oil
1 teaspoon unsalted butter
½ sweet onion, chopped
4 cups chopped watercress
¼ cup chopped fresh parsley
3 cups water
¼ cup heavy cream
1 tablespoon freshly squeezed lemon juice
Freshly ground black pepper

1. Preheat the oven to 400°F.
2. Place the garlic on a piece of aluminum foil. Drizzle with olive oil and fold the foil into a little packet. Place the packet in a pie plate and roast the garlic for about 20 minutes or until very soft.
3. Remove the garlic from the oven; set aside to cool.
4. In a large saucepan over medium-high heat, melt the butter. Sauté the onion for about 4 minutes or until soft. Add the watercress and parsley; sauté 5 minutes.
5. Stir in the water and roasted garlic pulp. Bring the soup to a boil, then reduce the heat to low.
6. Simmer the soup for about 20 minutes or until the vegetables are soft.
7. Cool the soup for about 5 minutes, then purée in batches in a food processor (or use a large bowl and a handheld immersion blender), along with the heavy cream.
8. Transfer the soup to the pot, and set over low heat until warmed through.
9. Add the lemon juice and season with pepper.

PER SERVING Calories: 97; Fat: 8g; Carbohydrates: 5g; Phosphorus: 46mg; Potassium: 198mg; Sodium: 23mg; Protein: 2g

CURRIED CAULIFLOWER SOUP

Serves 6 / Prep time: 20 minutes / Cook time: 30 minutes

Cauliflower is a cruciferous vegetable that is often used to provide bulk and texture to recipes. This vegetable also soaks up flavors easily, so it is a logical choice for a curried soup. Cauliflower is full of antioxidants, fiber, and B vitamins, and offers many health benefits, including decreasing the risk of cancer, heart disease, and other inflammatory diseases.

1 teaspoon unsalted butter
1 small sweet onion, chopped
2 teaspoons minced garlic
1 small head cauliflower, cut into small florets
3 cups water, or more to cover the cauliflower
2 teaspoons curry powder
½ cup light sour cream
3 tablespoons chopped fresh cilantro

1. In a large saucepan, heat the butter over medium-high heat and sauté the onion and garlic for about 3 minutes or until softened.

2. Add the cauliflower, water, and curry powder.

3. Bring the soup to a boil, then reduce the heat to low and simmer for about 20 minutes or until the cauliflower is tender.

4. Pour the soup into a food processor and purée until the soup is smooth and creamy (or use a large bowl and a handheld immersion blender).

5. Transfer the soup back into a saucepan and stir in the sour cream and cilantro.

6. Heat the soup on medium-low for about 5 minutes or until warmed through.

PER SERVING Calories: 33; Fat: 2g; Carbohydrates: 4g; Phosphorus: 30mg; Potassium: 167mg; Sodium: 22mg; Protein: 1g

ROASTED RED PEPPER AND EGGPLANT SOUP

Serves 6 / Prep time: 20 minutes / Cook time: 40 minutes

The process to create this soup may seem odd to you at first, but the results are delightful. Roast the vegetables first and then create the desired soup thickness by blending the finished vegetables with chicken stock. Use homemade chicken stock in your recipes or a carefully vetted commercial product to avoid consuming too much potassium and sodium.

1 small sweet onion, cut into quarters
2 small red bell peppers, halved
2 cups cubed eggplant
2 garlic cloves, crushed
1 tablespoon olive oil
1 cup Easy Chicken Stock (page 77)
Water
¼ cup chopped fresh basil
Freshly ground black pepper

1. Preheat the oven to 350°F.
2. Put the onions, red peppers, eggplant, and garlic in a large ovenproof baking dish.
3. Drizzle the vegetables with the olive oil.
4. Roast the vegetables for about 30 minutes or until they are slightly charred and soft.
5. Cool the vegetables slightly and remove the skin from the peppers.
6. Purée the vegetables in batches in a food processor (or in a large bowl, using a handheld immersion blender) with the chicken stock.
7. Transfer the soup to a medium pot and add enough water to reach the desired thickness. Heat the soup to a simmer and add the basil.
8. Season with pepper and serve.

PER SERVING Calories: 61; Fat: 2g; Carbohydrates: 9g; Phosphorus: 33mg; Potassium: 198mg; Sodium: 95mg; Protein: 2g

TRADITIONAL CHICKEN-VEGETABLE SOUP

Serves 6 / Prep time: 20 minutes / Cook time: 35 minutes

This classic cure for the common cold is a staple soup in many homes. Almost any ingredient works well with this basic recipe, and it freezes well, so make a double batch when you want an easy meal.

1 tablespoon unsalted butter

½ sweet onion, diced

2 teaspoons minced garlic

2 celery stalks, chopped

1 carrot, diced

2 cups chopped cooked chicken breast

1 cup Easy Chicken Stock (page 77)

4 cups water

1 teaspoon chopped fresh thyme

Freshly ground black pepper

2 tablespoons chopped fresh parsley

1. In a large pot over medium heat, melt the butter.

2. Sauté the onion and garlic until softened, about 3 minutes.

3. Add the celery, carrot, chicken, chicken stock, and water.

4. Bring the soup to a boil, reduce the heat, and simmer for about 30 minutes or until the vegetables are tender.

5. Add the thyme; simmer the soup for 2 minutes.

6. Season with pepper and serve topped with parsley.

PER SERVING Calories: 121; Fat: 6g; Carbohydrates: 2g; Phosphorus: 108mg; Potassium: 199mg; Sodium: 62mg; Protein: 15g

TURKEY-BULGUR SOUP

Serves 6 / Prep time: 25 minutes / Cook time: 45 minutes

Turkey may be an overlooked ingredient because chicken seems more available in stores. Turkey is a wonderful, healthy choice for this soup because it is high in protein, zinc, and iron and low in saturated fat. Try to purchase organic, pasture-raised turkey when possible.

1 teaspoon olive oil
½ pound cooked ground turkey, 93% lean
½ sweet onion, chopped
1 teaspoon minced garlic
4 cups water
1 cup Easy Chicken Stock (page 77)
1 celery stalk, chopped
1 carrot, sliced thin
½ cup shredded green cabbage
½ cup bulgur
2 dried bay leaves
2 tablespoons chopped fresh parsley
1 teaspoon chopped fresh sage
1 teaspoon chopped fresh thyme
Pinch red pepper flakes
Freshly ground black pepper

1. Place a large saucepan over medium-high heat and add the olive oil. Sauté the turkey for about 5 minutes or until the meat is cooked through.

2. Add the onion and garlic and sauté for about 3 minutes or until the vegetables are softened. Add the water, chicken stock, celery, carrot, cabbage, bulgur, and bay leaves.

3. Bring the soup to a boil and then reduce the heat to low and simmer for about 35 minutes or until the bulgur and vegetables are tender.

4. Remove the bay leaves and stir in the parsley, sage, thyme, and red pepper flakes.

5. Season with pepper and serve.

PER SERVING Calories: 77; Fat: 4g; Carbohydrates: 2g; Phosphorus: 82mg; Potassium: 175mg; Sodium: 54mg; Protein: 8g

GROUND BEEF AND RICE SOUP

Serves 6 / Prep time: 15 minutes / Cook time: 40 minutes

Try not to break up the ground beef completely when cooking because chunks create a nice texture. For an interesting variation, mix the ground beef with a few tablespoons of bread crumbs, garlic powder, and thyme, and roll the mixture into small meatballs. When the soup is simmering, drop in the meatballs and simmer for about 30 minutes, until they are cooked through.

½ pound extra-lean ground beef
½ small sweet onion, chopped
1 teaspoon minced garlic
2 cups water
1 cup homemade low-sodium beef broth
½ cup long-grain white rice, uncooked
1 celery stalk, chopped
½ cup fresh green beans, cut into 1-inch pieces
1 teaspoon chopped fresh thyme
Freshly ground black pepper

1. Place a large saucepan over medium-high heat and add the ground beef.
2. Sauté, stirring often, for about 6 minutes or until the beef is completely browned.
3. Drain off the excess fat and add the onion and garlic to the saucepan.
4. Sauté the vegetables for about 3 minutes or until they are softened.
5. Add the water, beef broth, rice, and celery.
6. Bring the soup to a boil, reduce the heat to low, and simmer for about 30 minutes or until the rice is tender.
7. Add the green beans and thyme and simmer for 3 minutes.
8. Remove the soup from the heat and season with pepper.

PER SERVING   Calories: 154; Fat: 7g; Carbohydrates: 14g; Phosphorus: 76mg; Potassium: 179mg; Sodium: 133mg; Protein: 9g

HERBED CABBAGE STEW

Serves 6 / Prep time: 20 minutes / Cook time: 35 minutes

Cabbage stew is a rustic, filling, low-calorie dish that takes little time to make and gets better while sitting in the refrigerator. This recipe produces a pretty green-hued stew with a subtle herb broth. The cabbage will soften and soak up the flavors, so add a little splash of hot sauce or a spoon of pesto for bolder flavor.

1 teaspoon unsalted butter
½ large sweet onion, chopped
1 teaspoon minced garlic
6 cups shredded green cabbage
3 celery stalks, chopped with the leafy tops
1 scallion, both green and white parts, chopped
2 tablespoons chopped fresh parsley
2 tablespoons freshly squeezed lemon juice
1 tablespoon chopped fresh thyme
1 teaspoon chopped savory
1 teaspoon chopped fresh oregano
Water
1 cup fresh green beans, cut into 1-inch pieces
Freshly ground black pepper

1. In a medium stockpot over medium-high heat, melt the butter.
2. Sauté the onion and garlic in the melted butter for about 3 minutes or until the vegetables are softened.
3. Add the cabbage, celery, scallion, parsley, lemon juice, thyme, savory, and oregano to the pot, and add enough water to cover the vegetables by about 4 inches.
4. Bring the soup to a boil, reduce the heat to low, and simmer the soup for about 25 minutes or until the vegetables are tender.
5. Add the green beans and simmer 3 minutes.
6. Season with pepper.

PER SERVING Calories: 33; Fat: 1g; Carbohydrates: 6g; Phosphorus: 29mg; Potassium: 187mg; Sodium: 20mg; Protein: 1g

WINTER CHICKEN STEW

Serves 6 / Prep time: 20 minutes / Cook time: 50 minutes

Stew is comfort food you may enjoy most during the cold winter, but you can certainly enjoy this stew in other seasons, too. If you prefer, make it in a slow cooker set on low for 10 hours. Simply brown the chicken breast and add it to all the other ingredients, except the cornstarch, in the slow cooker. Stir in the cornstarch when the stew is done if you need to thicken the sauce.

1 tablespoon olive oil

1 pound boneless, skinless chicken thighs, cut into 1-inch cubes

½ sweet onion, chopped

1 tablespoon minced garlic

2 cups Easy Chicken Stock (page 77)

1 cup plus 2 tablespoons water

1 carrot, sliced

2 celery stalks, sliced

1 turnip, sliced thin

1 tablespoon chopped fresh thyme

1 teaspoon finely chopped fresh rosemary

2 teaspoons cornstarch

Freshly ground black pepper

1. Place a large saucepan on medium-high heat and add the olive oil.

2. Sauté the chicken for about 6 minutes or until it is lightly browned, stirring often.

3. Add the onion and garlic and sauté for 3 minutes.

4. Add the chicken stock, 1 cup water, carrot, celery, and turnip and bring the stew to a boil.

5. Reduce the heat to low and simmer for about 30 minutes or until the chicken is cooked through and tender.

6. Add the thyme and rosemary and simmer for 3 more minutes.

7. In a small bowl, stir together the 2 tablespoons water and the cornstarch, and add the mixture to the stew.

8. Stir to incorporate the cornstarch mixture and cook for 3 to 4 minutes or until the stew thickens.

9. Remove from the heat and season with pepper.

PER SERVING Calories: 141; Fat: 8g; Carbohydrates: 5g; Phosphorus: 53mg; Potassium: 192mg; Sodium: 214mg; Protein: 9g

ROASTED BEEF STEW

Serves 6 / Prep time: 30 minutes / Cook time: 1 hour, 15 minutes

Stew is a very economical dish because it uses inexpensive cuts of beef. These inexpensive cuts are tougher but very flavorful, and they benefit from long cooking times. Roasting the stew in the oven provides the perfect moist environment and timing to produce fork-tender meat.

¼ cup all-purpose flour
1 teaspoon freshly ground black pepper, plus extra for seasoning
Pinch cayenne pepper
½ pound boneless beef chuck roast, trimmed of fat and cut into 1-inch chunks
2 tablespoons olive oil
½ sweet onion, chopped
2 teaspoons minced garlic
1 cup homemade beef stock
1 cup plus 2 tablespoons water
1 carrot, cut into ½-inch chunks
2 celery stalks, chopped with greens
1 teaspoon chopped fresh thyme
1 teaspoon cornstarch
2 tablespoons chopped fresh parsley

1. Preheat the oven to 350°F.
2. Put the flour, black pepper, and cayenne pepper in a large plastic freezer bag and toss to mix.
3. Add the beef chunks to the bag and toss to coat.
4. In a large ovenproof pot, heat the olive oil.
5. Sauté the beef chunks for about 5 minutes or until they are lightly browned. Remove the beef from the pot and set aside on a plate.
6. Add the onion and garlic to the pot and sauté for 3 minutes.
7. Stir in the beef stock and deglaze the pot, scraping up any bits on the bottom.

8. Add 1 cup water, the beef drippings on the plate, the carrot, celery, and thyme.

9. Cover the pot tightly with a lid or aluminum foil and place in the oven.

10. Bake the stew, stirring occasionally, for about 1 hour or until the meat is very tender.

11. Remove the stew from the oven.

12. In a small bowl, stir together the 2 tablespoons water and the cornstarch and then stir the mixture into the hot stew to thicken the sauce.

13. Season the stew with black pepper and serve topped with parsley.

PER SERVING Calories: 163; Fat: 10g; Carbohydrates: 7g; Phosphorus: 89mg; Potassium: 200mg; Sodium: 121mg; Protein: 11g

CHAPTER TEN

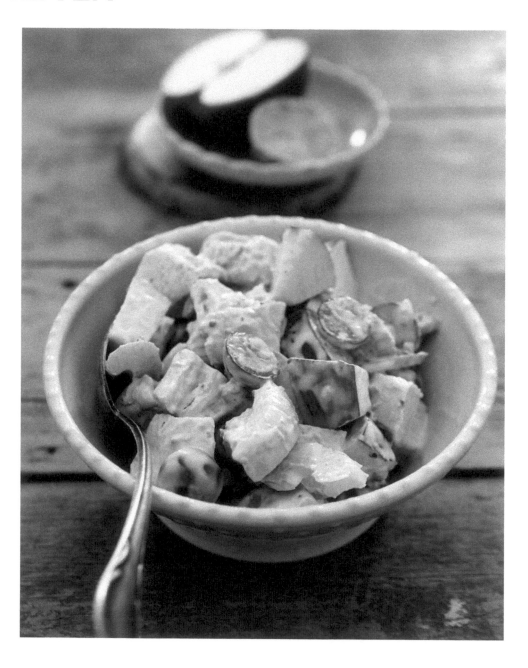

SALADS

LEAF LETTUCE AND CARROT SALAD WITH BALSAMIC VINAIGRETTE

Serves 4 / Prep time: 25 minutes

A simple salad combined with flavorful vinaigrette is a wonderful starter or light meal when topped with a piece of broiled fish or grilled chicken. You can easily make more of the vinaigrette recipe if you want to keep some dressing on hand. Add all the vinaigrette ingredients to a mason jar and shake it up whenever you need it.

FOR THE VINAIGRETTE

½ cup olive oil

4 tablespoons balsamic vinegar

2 tablespoons chopped fresh oregano

Pinch red pepper flakes

Freshly ground black pepper

FOR THE SALAD

4 cups shredded green leaf lettuce

1 carrot, shredded

¾ cup fresh green beans, cut into 1-inch pieces

3 large radishes, sliced thin

TO MAKE THE VINAIGRETTE

1. In a small bowl, whisk together the olive oil, balsamic vinegar, oregano, and red pepper flakes.

2. Season with pepper.

TO MAKE THE SALAD

1. In a large bowl, toss together the lettuce, carrot, green beans, and radishes.

2. Add the vinaigrette to the vegetables and toss to coat.

3. Arrange the salad on 4 plates to serve.

PER SERVING Calories: 273; Fat: 27g; Carbohydrates: 7g; Phosphorus: 30mg; Potassium: 197mg; Sodium: 27mg; Protein: 1g

STRAWBERRY-WATERCRESS SALAD WITH ALMOND DRESSING

Serves 6 / Prep time: 15 minutes

Fresh, ripe strawberries add a splash of vivid color and sweetness to this salad, and the almond dressing is an unexpected twist. Strawberries are packed with nutrients—they are an excellent source of vitamin C, folate, and fiber, and they are among the top 20 fruits in disease-fighting antioxidants. They can increase your good (HDL) cholesterol and lower your blood pressure, which means they may be good for your heart in more ways than one.

FOR THE DRESSING

¼ cup olive oil

¼ cup rice vinegar

1 tablespoon honey

¼ teaspoon pure almond extract

¼ teaspoon ground mustard

Freshly ground black pepper

FOR THE SALAD

2 cups roughly chopped watercress

2 cups shredded green leaf lettuce

½ red onion, sliced very thin

½ English cucumber, chopped

1 cup sliced strawberries

TO MAKE THE DRESSING

1. In a small bowl, whisk together the olive oil and rice vinegar until emulsified.

2. Whisk in the honey, almond extract, mustard, and pepper; set aside.

TO MAKE THE SALAD

1. In a large bowl, toss together the watercress, green leaf lettuce, onion, cucumber, and strawberries.

2. Pour the dressing over the salad and toss to combine.

PER SERVING Calories: 159; Fat: 14g; Carbohydrates: 9g; Phosphorus: 34mg; Potassium: 195mg; Sodium: 14mg; Protein: 1g

CUCUMBER-DILL CABBAGE SALAD WITH LEMON DRESSING

Serves 4 / Prep time: 25 minutes, plus 1 hour to chill

The wonderfully crunchy cucumber is filled with cool, refreshing juice, making it a natural, mild diuretic. After you slice the cucumber for this recipe, let it sit for 30 minutes to allow the liquid to be released from the slices. Pour off the liquid before mixing in the other ingredients. Most of the nutrition in cucumbers is found in the skin, so scrub it carefully and leave it on whenever a recipe permits. Cucumbers are a good source of vitamin A, vitamin C, and beta-carotene.

¼ cup heavy cream
¼ cup freshly squeezed lemon juice
2 tablespoons granulated sugar
2 tablespoons chopped fresh dill
2 tablespoons finely chopped scallion, green part only
¼ teaspoon freshly ground black pepper
1 English cucumber, sliced thin
2 cups shredded green cabbage

1. In a small bowl, stir together the cream, lemon juice, sugar, dill, scallion, and pepper until well blended.

2. In a large bowl, toss together the cucumber and cabbage.

3. Place the salad in the refrigerator and chill for 1 hour.

4. Stir before serving.

PER SERVING Calories: 99; Fat: 6g; Carbohydrates: 13g; Phosphorus: 38mg; Potassium: 200mg; Sodium: 14mg: Protein: 2g

LEAF LETTUCE AND ASPARAGUS SALAD WITH RASPBERRIES

Serves 4 / Prep time: 25 minutes

The asparagus in this recipe is raw and prepared in pretty, pale ribbons that curl around the other ingredients. Centuries ago, asparagus was considered a medicinal vegetable, especially with respect to the kidneys and bladder. Asparagus acts as a natural diuretic, and it is a good source of fiber, folate, iron, and vitamins A, C, E, and K.

2 cups shredded green leaf lettuce
1 cup asparagus, cut into long ribbons with a peeler
1 scallion, both green and white parts, sliced
1 cup raspberries
2 tablespoons balsamic vinegar
Freshly ground black pepper

1. Arrange the lettuce evenly on 4 serving plates.

2. Arrange the asparagus and scallion on top of the greens.

3. Place the raspberries on top of the salads, dividing the berries evenly.

4. Drizzle the salads with balsamic vinegar.

5. Season with pepper.

PER SERVING Calories: 36; Fat: 0g; Carbohydrates: 8g; Phosphorus: 43mg; Potassium: 200mg; Sodium: 11mg; Protein: 2g

WALDORF SALAD

Serves 4 / Prep time: 20 minutes

Waldorf salad was created in 1893 by the maître d'hôtel of the Waldorf Astoria in New York City. That original salad did not use a sour cream dressing and contained walnuts. This adaption is as spectacular as the original, and it can be topped with diced chicken if you need more protein in your diet.

3 cups green leaf lettuce, torn into pieces

1 cup halved grapes

3 celery stalks, chopped

1 large apple, cored, peeled, and chopped

½ cup light sour cream

2 tablespoons freshly squeezed lemon juice

1 tablespoon granulated sugar

1. Arrange the lettuce evenly on 4 plates; set aside.

2. In a small bowl, stir together the grapes, celery, and apple.

3. In another small bowl, stir together the sour cream, lemon juice, and sugar.

4. Add the sour cream mixture to the grape mixture and stir to coat.

5. Spoon the dressed grape mixture onto each plate, dividing the mixture evenly.

PER SERVING Calories: 73; Fat: 2g; Carbohydrates: 15g; Phosphorus: 29mg; Potassium: 194mg; Sodium: 30mg; Protein: 1g

ASIAN PEAR SALAD

Serves 6 / Prep time: 30 minutes, plus 1 hour to chill

Asian pears are the pale, round fruit wrapped protectively in a lacy slipcover and are found in the grocery store next to the regular pears. They look fragile but grate easily for this salad without getting mushy. These juicy, firm-textured pears add crisp sweetness to the vegetables in this slaw. You can substitute regular pears if you can't find Asian pears in your local store.

2 cups finely shredded green cabbage

1 cup finely shredded red cabbage

2 scallions, both green and white parts, chopped

2 celery stalks, chopped

1 Asian pear, cored and grated

½ red bell pepper, boiled and chopped

½ cup chopped cilantro

¼ cup olive oil

Juice of 1 lime

Zest of 1 lime

1 teaspoon granulated sugar

1. In a large bowl, toss together the green and red cabbage, scallions, celery, pear, red pepper, and cilantro.

2. In a small bowl, whisk together the olive oil, lime juice, lime zest, and sugar.

3. Add the dressing to the cabbage mixture and toss to combine.

4. Chill for 1 hour in the refrigerator before serving.

PER SERVING Calories: 105; Fat: 9g; Carbohydrates: 6g; Phosphorus: 17mg; Potassium: 136mg; Sodium: 48mg; Protein: 1g

COUSCOUS SALAD WITH SPICY CITRUS DRESSING

Serves 6 / Prep time: 25 minutes, plus 1 hour to chill

Couscous looks like a whole grain, but it is pasta made from semolina wheat that is steamed to a tender finish. Couscous is an ingredient found in many recipes in North Africa, and it is traditionally served topped with a meat or vegetable stew. It pairs wonderfully with a variety of flavors as a main dish, side dish, or salad.

FOR THE DRESSING

¼ cup olive oil

3 tablespoons freshly squeezed grapefruit juice

Juice of 1 lime

Zest of 1 lime

1 tablespoon chopped fresh parsley

Pinch cayenne pepper

Freshly ground black pepper

FOR THE SALAD

3 cups cooked couscous, chilled

½ red bell pepper, chopped

1 scallion, both white and green parts, chopped

1 apple, cored and chopped

TO MAKE THE DRESSING

1. In a small bowl, whisk together the olive oil, grapefruit juice, lime juice, lime zest, parsley, and cayenne pepper.

2. Season with black pepper.

TO MAKE THE SALAD

1. In a large bowl, mix together the chilled couscous, red pepper, scallion, and apple.

2. Add the dressing to the couscous mixture and toss to combine.

3. Chill in the refrigerator for at least 1 hour before serving.

Substitution tip: *If you are taking a medication that prevents you from eating grapefruit, you can substitute any citrus juice, like lemon, lime, or tangerine, for grapefruit juice.*

PER SERVING Calories: 187; Fat: 9g; Carbohydrates: 23g; Phosphorus: 24mg; Potassium: 108mg; Sodium: 5mg; Protein: 3g

FARFALLE CONFETTI SALAD

Serves 6 / Prep time: 30 minutes, plus 1 hour to chill

If you have a picnic or barbecue to attend, whip up this colorful dish and tote it along. The red, green, orange, and yellow vegetable flecks look pretty against the light-hued pasta and creamy dressing. Add some freshly chopped chives and a teaspoon of lemon zest as garnishes if you want an elegant finish.

2 cups cooked farfalle pasta
¼ cup boiled and finely chopped red bell pepper
¼ cup finely chopped cucumber
¼ cup grated carrot
2 tablespoons yellow bell pepper
½ scallion, green part only, finely chopped
½ cup Homemade Mayonnaise (page 71)
1 tablespoon freshly squeezed lemon juice
1 teaspoon chopped fresh parsley
½ teaspoon granulated sugar
Freshly ground black pepper

1. In a large bowl, toss together the pasta, red pepper, cucumber, carrot, yellow pepper, and scallion.

2. In a small bowl, whisk together the mayonnaise, lemon juice, parsley, and sugar.

3. Add the dressing to the pasta mixture and stir to combine.

4. Season with pepper.

5. Chill in the refrigerator for at least 1 hour before serving.

PER SERVING Calories: 119; Fat: 3g; Carbohydrates: 20g; Phosphorus: 51mg; Potassium: 82mg; Sodium: 16mg; Protein: 4g

TABBOULEH

Serves 6 / Prep time: 30 minutes, plus 1 hour to chill

Traditional tabbouleh features heaps of chopped herbs, usually mint, and it can be made with bulgur instead of couscous. The dressing is very simple—just a splash of olive oil and lemon juice. So use fresh juice and good-quality oil for the best results. This salad is best if it sits in the refrigerator for at least 1 hour to allow the flavors to deepen.

4 cups cooked white rice
½ red bell pepper, boiled and finely chopped
½ yellow bell pepper, boiled and chopped
½ zucchini, finely chopped, boiled until tender
1 cup chopped eggplant, boiled until tender
¼ cup finely chopped fresh parsley
¼ cup finely chopped fresh cilantro
2 tablespoons olive oil
Juice of 1 lemon
Zest of 1 lemon
Freshly ground black pepper

1. In a large bowl, stir together the rice, red bell pepper, yellow bell pepper, zucchini, eggplant, parsley, cilantro, olive oil, lemon juice, and lemon zest until well combined.

2. Season with pepper.

3. Chill the salad in the refrigerator for at least 1 hour before serving.

PER SERVING Calories: 177; Fat: 5g; Carbohydrates: 29g; Phosphorus: 46mg; Potassium: 189mg; Sodium: 78mg; Protein: 4g

GINGER BEEF SALAD

Serves 6 / Prep time: 30 minutes, plus 1 hour to marinate / Cook time: 10 minutes

Men love this salad. It is simple, uses hot radishes and robust red onions, and sports a topping of juicy grilled beef. The beef marinade in this recipe is very spicy, so if you prefer a milder flavor, omit the chili paste. If you don't have a barbecue, the meat can be broiled for 6 minutes per side in the oven instead.

FOR THE BEEF

2 tablespoons olive oil

2 tablespoons freshly squeezed lime juice

1 tablespoon grated fresh ginger

2 teaspoons minced garlic

½ pound flank steak

FOR THE VINAIGRETTE

¼ cup olive oil

¼ cup rice vinegar

Juice of 1 lime

Zest of 1 lime

1 tablespoon honey

1 teaspoon chopped fresh thyme

FOR THE SALAD

4 cups torn green leaf lettuce

½ red onion, sliced thin

½ cup sliced radishes

TO MAKE THE BEEF

1. In a small bowl, stir together the olive oil, lime juice, ginger, and garlic until well blended.

2. Add the flank steak to the marinade and turn it to coat both sides of the meat.

3. Cover the bowl with plastic wrap and place in the refrigerator for 1 hour to marinate.

4. Remove the steak from the marinade and discard the marinade.

5. Preheat a barbecue to medium-high and grill the steak to medium doneness, turning once, for about 5 minutes per side, depending on the thickness of the steak.

6. Remove the steak; place on a cutting board and let the meat rest for 10 minutes.

7. Slicing the meat thinly across the grain.

TO MAKE THE VINAIGRETTE

In a small bowl, whisk together the olive oil, rice vinegar, lime juice, lime zest, honey, and thyme; set aside.

TO MAKE THE SALAD

1. Arrange the lettuce, onion, and radishes on 6 plates, dividing evenly.

2. Drizzle each salad with vinaigrette.

3. Top each salad with the sliced beef.

PER SERVING Calories: 200; Fat: 14g; Carbohydrates: 5g; Phosphorus: 84mg; Potassium: 193mg; Sodium: 29mg; Protein: 8g

CHAPTER ELEVEN

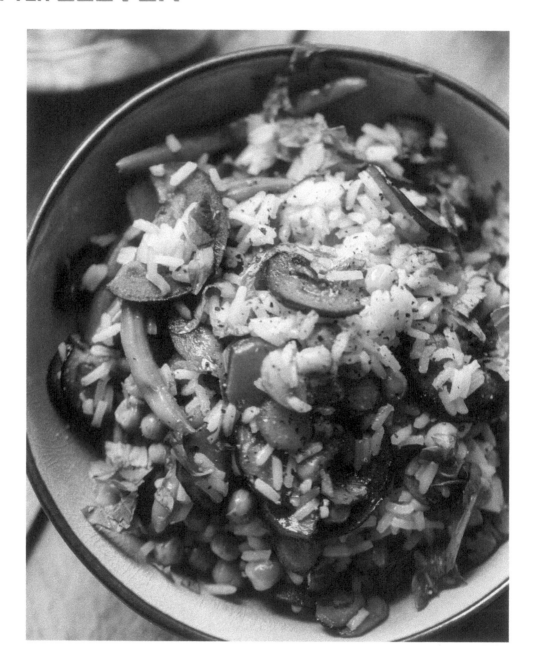

VEGETARIAN ENTRÉES

EGG WHITE FRITTATA WITH PENNE

Serves 4 / Prep time: 15 minutes / Cook time: 30 minutes

A frittata is one of the easiest ways to prepare eggs, and the results look like you've spent hours in the kitchen. Even if you make frittatas all the time, adding pasta may be a new twist. Pasta creates a heartier dish that is perfect for lunch on a busy weekend or cut up into squares for a road trip.

6 egg whites
¼ cup rice milk
1 tablespoon chopped fresh parsley
1 teaspoon chopped fresh thyme
1 teaspoon chopped fresh chives
Freshly ground black pepper
2 teaspoons olive oil
¼ small sweet onion, chopped
1 teaspoon minced garlic
½ cup boiled and chopped red bell pepper
2 cups cooked penne

1. Preheat the oven to 350°F.
2. In a large bowl, whisk together the egg whites, rice milk, parsley, thyme, chives, and pepper.
3. In a large ovenproof skillet over medium heat, heat the olive oil.
4. Sauté the onion, garlic, and red pepper for about 4 minutes or until they are softened.
5. Using a spatula, add the cooked penne to the skillet to evenly distribute the pasta.
6. Pour the egg mixture over the pasta and shake the pan to coat the pasta.
7. Leave the skillet on the heat for 1 minute to set the bottom of the frittata and then transfer the skillet to the oven.
8. Bake the frittata for about 25 minutes or until it is set and golden brown.
9. Remove from the oven and serve immediately.

PER SERVING   Calories: 170; Fat: 3g; Carbohydrates: 25g; Phosphorus: 62mg; Potassium: 144mg; Sodium: 90mg; Protein: 10g

VEGETABLE FRIED RICE

Serves 6 / Prep time: 20 minutes / Cook time: 20 minutes

If you find fried rice in restaurants is too greasy and salty, this fresh, flavorful dish will be a satisfying treat. For a more substantial dish, add two beaten eggs scrambled right in the pan at the end. Push the rice and vegetables aside, creating an empty spot in the skillet, and scramble the eggs before stirring them back into the rice mixture. This will add about 30 mg of phosphorus and 20 mg of potassium to each serving.

1 tablespoon olive oil

½ sweet onion, chopped

1 tablespoon grated fresh ginger

2 teaspoons minced garlic

1 cup sliced carrots

½ cup chopped eggplant

½ cup peas

½ cup green beans, cut into 1-inch pieces

2 tablespoons chopped fresh cilantro

3 cups cooked rice

1. In a large skillet over medium-high heat, heat the olive oil.
2. Sauté the onion, ginger, and garlic for about 3 minutes or until softened.
3. Stir in the carrot, eggplant, peas, and green beans and sauté for 3 minutes more.
4. Add the cilantro and rice.
5. Sauté, stirring constantly, for about 10 minutes or until the rice is heated through.
6. Serve immediately.

PER SERVING Calories: 189; Fat: 7g; Carbohydrates: 28g; Phosphorus: 89mg; Potassium: 172mg; Sodium: 13mg; Protein: 6g

BULGUR-STUFFED SPAGHETTI SQUASH

Serves 4 / Prep time: 20 minutes / Cook time: 50 minutes

Golden squash makes a convenient and pretty container to hold vegetables, grains, spices, and fruit. The most important part of creating this meal is to make sure you don't pierce the skin while scooping out the roasted flesh. A hole in the squash shell will allow the juices and filling to escape.

FOR THE SQUASH

2 small spaghetti squash, halved

1 teaspoon olive oil

Freshly ground black pepper

FOR THE FILLING

1 teaspoon olive oil

½ small sweet onion, finely diced

1 teaspoon minced garlic

½ cup chopped carrot

½ cup cranberries

1 teaspoon chopped fresh thyme

½ teaspoon ground cumin

½ teaspoon ground coriander

Juice of ½ lemon

1 cup cooked bulgur

TO MAKE THE SQUASH

1. Preheat the oven to 350°F.

2. Line a baking sheet with parchment paper.

3. Lightly oil the cut sides of the squash, season with pepper, and place them cut-side down on the baking sheet.

4. Bake for 25 to 30 minutes or until tender. Remove the squash from the oven and flip the squash halves over.

5. Scoop out the flesh from each half, leaving about ½ inch around the edges and keeping the skin intact.

6. Place 2 cups of squash flesh in a large bowl and reserve the rest for another recipe.

TO MAKE THE FILLING

1. In a medium skillet over medium heat, heat the olive oil.

2. Sauté the onion, garlic, carrot, and cranberries for 5 to 6 minutes or until softened.

3. Add the sautéed vegetables to the squash in the bowl.

4. Add the thyme, cumin, and coriander, stirring to combine.

5. Stir in the lemon juice and cooked bulgur until well mixed.

6. Spoon the filling evenly into the squash halves.

7. Bake in the oven for about 15 minutes or until heated through.

8. Serve warm.

PER SERVING Calories: 111; Fat: 2g; Carbohydrates: 17g; Phosphorus: 38mg; Potassium: 182mg; Sodium: 22mg; Protein: 3g

RED PEPPER STRATA

Serves 8 / Prep time: 20 minutes, plus 2 hours soaking time /
Cook time: 1 hour, 5 minutes

Centuries ago, savory bread pudding was a tasty way to use up stale bread, leftovers, and eggs when serving large groups of people. This dish can be doubled easily, other vegetables can be added, and it can be prepared the night before for convenience. If you want enhanced flavor, use a homemade, herb-infused vinegar.

Butter, for greasing the baking dish
8 slices fresh white bread, cut into cubes
1 tablespoon unsalted butter
½ sweet onion, chopped
1 teaspoon minced garlic
1 red bell pepper, boiled and chopped
6 eggs
¼ cup tarragon vinegar
1 cup rice milk
1 teaspoon Tabasco sauce
½ teaspoon freshly ground black pepper
1 ounce Parmesan cheese, grated

1. Preheat the oven to 250°F.
2. Lightly grease a 9-by-9-inch baking dish with butter; set aside.
3. Line a baking sheet with parchment paper and scatter the bread cubes on the sheet.
4. Bake the bread cubes for about 10 minutes or until they are crisp.
5. Remove the bread cubes from the oven; set aside.
6. In a medium skillet over medium-high heat, melt the butter.
7. Sauté the onion and garlic for about 3 minutes or until softened.
8. Add the red pepper and sauté an additional 2 minutes.

9. Spread half of the bread cubes in a layer in the baking dish and top with half of the sautéed vegetables.

10. Repeat with the remaining half of the bread cubes and vegetables.

11. In a medium bowl, whisk together the eggs, vinegar, rice milk, hot sauce, and pepper.

12. Pour the egg mixture evenly into the baking dish.

13. Cover the dish and place in the fridge to soak for at least 2 hours or overnight.

14. Let the strata come to room temperature.

15. Preheat the oven to 325°F.

16. Remove the plastic wrap and bake for about 45 minutes or until golden.

17. Sprinkle the top of the strata with cheese and bake an additional 5 minutes.

18. Serve hot.

PER SERVING Calories: 150; Fat: 6g; Carbohydrates: 10g; Phosphorus: 120mg; Potassium: 89mg; Sodium: 168mg; Protein: 7g

COUSCOUS BURGERS

Serves 4 / Prep time: 20 minutes, plus 1 hour chilling time / Cook time: 10 minutes

Veggie burgers have a bad reputation because they are often tasteless and dry or have a strange texture. Couscous is a delightfully tender base, especially when infused with citrus and herbs. You can make a double batch and freeze the uncooked patties for up to 3 months for a quick and convenient meal. Serve them alone or on a bun with your favorite toppings.

½ cup canned chickpeas, rinsed and drained

2 tablespoons chopped fresh cilantro

2 tablespoons chopped fresh parsley

1 tablespoon freshly squeezed lemon juice

2 teaspoons lemon zest

1 teaspoon minced garlic

2½ cups cooked couscous

2 eggs, lightly beaten

2 tablespoons olive oil

1. Put the chickpeas, cilantro, parsley, lemon juice, lemon zest, and garlic in a food processor and pulse until a paste forms (or use a large bowl and a handheld immersion blender).

2. Transfer the chickpea mixture to a bowl and add the couscous and eggs, mixing thoroughly to combine.

3. Chill the mixture in the refrigerator for 1 hour to firm it.

4. Form the couscous mixture into 4 patties.

5. Place a large skillet over medium-high heat and add the olive oil.

6. Place the patties in the skillet, 2 at a time, gently pressing them down with the back of a spatula. Cook for 5 minutes or until golden, and flip the patties over.

7. Cook the other side for 5 minutes and transfer the cooked burgers to a plate covered with a paper towel.

8. Repeat with the remaining 2 burgers.

PER SERVING Calories: 242; Fat: 10g; Carbohydrates: 29g; Phosphorus: 108mg; Potassium: 168mg; Sodium: 43mg; Protein: 9g

MARINATED TOFU STIR-FRY

Serves 4 / Prep time: 20 minutes, plus 2 hours chilling time / Cook time: 20 minutes

Tofu is an incredible ingredient that soaks up any flavors. It is a good source of protein and excellent source of calcium. Tofu is sold in different textures, from silken to extra-firm, so it can be used in many types of cuisine. Extra-firm tofu is best when you are marinating and stir-frying because it will hold its shape and not fall apart.

FOR THE TOFU

1 tablespoon freshly squeezed lemon juice

1 teaspoon minced garlic

1 teaspoon grated fresh ginger

Pinch red pepper flakes

5 ounces extra-firm tofu, pressed well and cubed (see ingredient tip)

FOR THE STIR-FRY

1 tablespoon olive oil

½ cup cauliflower florets

½ cup thinly sliced carrots

½ cup julienned red pepper

½ cup fresh green beans

2 cups cooked white rice

TO MAKE THE TOFU

1. In a small bowl, mix together the lemon juice, garlic, ginger, and red pepper flakes.

2. Add the tofu and toss to coat.

3. Place the bowl in the refrigerator and marinate for 2 hours. ▶

TO MAKE THE STIR FRY

1. In a large skillet over medium-high heat, heat the oil.

2. Sauté the tofu for about 8 minutes or until it is lightly browned and heated through.

3. Add the cauliflower and carrots and sauté for 5 minutes, stirring and tossing constantly.

4. Add the red pepper and green beans; sauté for 3 additional minutes.

5. Serve over the white rice.

Ingredient tip: *Draining tofu is a crucial step to ensure this porous product absorbs all the flavor in the dish. Place the tofu on a paper towel-lined plate and cover the block with more paper towels. Set something heavy such as a large can or a book on the tofu. Check the drainage every 30 minutes, changing the paper towels if needed, for two hours.*

Dialysis modification: *Omit the red peppers from the dish to lower the amount of potassium in the recipe.*

PER SERVING   Calories: 190; Fat: 6g; Carbohydrates: 30g; Phosphorus: 90mg; Potassium: 199mg; Sodium: 22mg; Protein: 6g

THAI-INSPIRED VEGETABLE CURRY

Serves 4 / Prep time: 15 minutes / Cook time: 45 minutes

Curry is a versatile dish that is equally at home in a fine-dining restaurant or eaten from a takeout box. This is because curry spices combine beautifully with many different ingredients, such as the eggplant, peppers, and carrots in this recipe. If you prefer a creamier sauce, add ¼ cup heavy (whipping) cream right at the end.

2 teaspoons olive oil

½ sweet onion, diced

2 teaspoons minced garlic

2 teaspoons grated fresh ginger

½ eggplant, peeled and diced

1 carrot, peeled and diced

1 red bell pepper, diced

1 tablespoon Hot Curry Powder (see page 87)

1 teaspoon ground cumin

½ teaspoon coriander

Pinch cayenne pepper

1½ cups homemade vegetable stock

1 tablespoon cornstarch

¼ cup water

1. In a large stockpot over medium-high heat, heat the oil.

2. Sauté the onion, garlic, and ginger for 3 minutes or until they are softened.

3. Add the eggplant, carrots, and red pepper, and sauté, stirring often, for 6 additional minutes.

4. Stir in the curry powder, cumin, coriander, cayenne pepper, and vegetable stock.

5. Bring the curry to a boil and then reduce the heat to low. ▶

6. Simmer the curry for about 30 minutes or until the vegetables are tender.

7. In a small bowl, stir together the cornstarch and water.

8. Stir the cornstarch mixture into the curry and simmer for about 5 minutes or until the sauce is thickened.

PER SERVING   Calories: 100; Fat: 3g; Carbohydrates: 9g; Phosphorus: 28mg; Potassium: 180mg; Sodium: 218mg; Protein: 1g

LINGUINE WITH ROASTED RED PEPPER–BASIL SAUCE

Serves 4 / Prep time: 20 minutes / Cook time: 20 minutes

Fresh basil imparts a wonderful aroma and flavor to this simple dish. This popular herb's oils and extracts are said to have antioxidant and antibacterial properties. Two of the vitamins it offers are vitamin A and blood-clotting vitamin K. When cooking with basil, add it to the dish at the end to retain the best color and maximum flavor.

8 ounces uncooked linguine

1 teaspoon olive oil

½ sweet onion, chopped

2 teaspoons minced garlic

1 cup chopped roasted red bell peppers

1 teaspoon balsamic vinegar

¼ cup shredded fresh basil

Pinch red pepper flakes

Freshly ground black pepper

4 teaspoons grated low-fat Parmesan cheese, for garnish

1. Cook the pasta according to the package instructions.

2. While the pasta is cooking, place a large skillet over medium-high heat and add the olive oil.

3. Sauté the onions and garlic for about 3 minutes or until they are softened.

4. Add the red pepper, vinegar, basil, and red pepper flakes to the skillet and stir for about 5 minutes or until heated through.

5. Toss the cooked pasta with the sauce and season with pepper.

6. Serve topped with Parmesan cheese.

PER SERVING Calories: 246; Fat: 3g; Carbohydrates: 41g; Phosphorus: 117mg; Potassium: 187mg; Sodium: 450mg; Protein: 13g

BAKED MAC AND CHEESE

Serves 4 / Prep time: 10 minutes / Cook time: 25 minutes

Creamy, rich, and cheesy is an accurate description of macaroni and cheese, but it doesn't have to be a guilty indulgence. This version has a hint of cayenne pepper, mustard, and garlic in the sauce, which adds a little heat in the background. Eat it immediately after cooking, because the sauce will become grainy if frozen and reheated.

Butter, for greasing the baking dish
1 teaspoon olive oil
½ sweet onion, chopped
1 teaspoon minced garlic
¼ cup rice milk
1 cup cream cheese
½ teaspoon dry mustard
½ teaspoon freshly ground black pepper
Pinch cayenne pepper
3 cups cooked macaroni

1. Preheat the oven to 375°F.
2. Grease a 9-by-9-inch baking dish with butter; set aside.
3. In a medium saucepan over medium heat, heat the olive oil.
4. Sauté the onion and garlic for about 3 minutes or until softened.
5. Stir in the milk, cheese, mustard, black pepper, and cayenne pepper until the mixture is smooth and well blended.
6. Add the cooked macaroni, stirring to coat.
7. Spoon the mixture into the baking dish and place in the oven.
8. Bake for about 15 minutes or until the macaroni is bubbly.

Dialysis modification: *This dish is rich, so you can choose a smaller portion size to reduce your phosphorus and potassium intake.*

PER SERVING Calories: 386; Fat: 22g; Carbohydrates: 37g; Phosphorus: 120mg; Potassium: 146mg; Sodium: 219mg; Protein: 10g

GRILLED KALE AND FRIED EGG ON BREAD

Serves 2 / Prep time: 10 minutes / Cook time: 20 minutes

A simple egg on a piece of toast becomes extraordinary with the addition of oven-crisped kale. This healthy green is packed with protein, fiber, and vitamins A, C, and K. It even offers some heart-healthy omega-3 fatty acids. When you buy kale at the supermarket, choose a bunch with dark, crisp leaves. When you cook with it, remove the ribs and toughest leaves first.

2 medium kale leaves
½ teaspoon olive oil
Pinch red pepper flakes
4 teaspoons unsalted butter, divided
2 slices white bread
2 teaspoons cream cheese
2 small eggs
Freshly ground black pepper

1. Preheat the oven to 350°F.
2. Massage the kale leaves with the olive oil until they are completely coated.
3. Sprinkle a pinch of red pepper flakes over the kale leaves.
4. Place the leaves in a pie plate and roast for about 10 minutes or until crispy.
5. Remove the kale from the oven; set aside.
6. Butter both sides of the bread with 1 teaspoon butter per slice.
7. In a large skillet over medium-high heat, toast the bread on both sides for about 3 minutes or until it is golden brown.
8. Remove the bread from the skillet and spread 1 teaspoon cream cheese on each slice. ▶

9. Melt the remaining 2 teaspoons of butter in the skillet and fry the eggs sunny-side up, for about 4 minutes.

10. Place a piece of crispy kale and a fried egg on top of each slice of the cream cheese-topped bread.

11. Serve seasoned with pepper.

PER SERVING   Calories: 224; Fat: 15g; Carbohydrates: 14g; Phosphorus: 118mg; Potassium: 175mg; Sodium: 200mg; Protein: 8g

TOFU AND EGGPLANT STIR-FRY

Serves 4 / Prep time: 20 minutes / Cook time: 20 minutes

Garlic, jalapeño, and ginger contribute to the intense flavor of the sauce in this recipe. Garlic has been shown to reduce the risk of heart disease and high blood pressure. It also may also protect against some cancers, fight inflammation, and give your immune system a boost. This recipe is delicious when served over rice or noodles.

1 tablespoon granulated sugar

1 tablespoon all-purpose flour

1 teaspoon grated fresh ginger

1 teaspoon minced garlic

1 teaspoon minced jalapeño pepper

Juice of 1 lime

Water

2 tablespoons olive oil, divided

5 ounces extra-firm tofu, cut into ½-inch cubes

2 cups cubed eggplant

2 scallions, both green and white parts, sliced

3 tablespoons chopped cilantro

1. In a small bowl, whisk together the sugar, flour, ginger, garlic, jalapeño, lime juice, and enough water to make ⅔ cup of sauce; set aside.

2. In a large skillet over medium-high heat, heat 1 tablespoon of the oil.

3. Sauté the tofu for about 6 minutes or until it is crisp and golden.

4. Remove the tofu; set aside on a plate.

5. Add the remaining 1 tablespoon oil and sauté the eggplant cubes for about 10 minutes or until they are fully cooked and lightly browned.

6. Add the tofu and scallions to the skillet and toss to combine.

7. Pour in the sauce and bring to a boil, stirring constantly, for about 2 minutes or until the sauce is thickened.

8. Add the cilantro before serving.

PER SERVING Calories: 386; Fat: 22g; Carbohydrates: 37g; Phosphorus: 120mg; Potassium: 146mg; Sodium: 219mg; Protein: 10g

MIE GORENG WITH BROCCOLI

Serves 4 / Prep time: 10 minutes, plus 30 minutes draining time / Cook time: 20 minutes

Indonesian food has complex flavors that stimulate the taste buds with salty, sweet, bitter, and spicy all at the same time. This dish includes sambal oelek, a spicy chile sauce from Southeast Asia. The word sambal *is Indonesian for a sauce made with green chiles, and* oelek *refers to the technique to make it using a mortar and pestle.*

½ pound rice noodles
¼ cup packed dark brown sugar
2 teaspoons minced garlic
1 teaspoon grated fresh ginger
1 teaspoon low-sodium soy sauce
½ teaspoon sambal oelek
4 ounces extra-firm tofu, cut into ½-inch cubes
1 tablespoon cornstarch
2 tablespoons olive oil, divided
2 cups broccoli, cut into small florets
2 scallions, both green and white parts, sliced thin on the diagonal
Lime wedges, for garnish

1. Cook the noodles according to the package instructions; drain and set aside.

2. In a small bowl, whisk together the brown sugar, garlic, ginger, soy sauce, and sambal oelek; set aside.

3. Drain the tofu on paper towels for 30 minutes and pat the tofu dry.

4. Toss the tofu with the cornstarch and shake to remove the excess.

5. In a large skillet over medium-high heat, heat 1 tablespoon of the olive oil.

6. Add the tofu and sauté for about 10 minutes or until the tofu is browned on all sides and crispy.

7. Transfer the tofu to a plate with a slotted spoon.

8. Add the remaining 1 tablespoon oil to the skillet.

9. Sauté the broccoli for about 4 minutes or until it is tender.

10. Add the sauce and tofu to the skillet and cook for about 2 minutes or until the sauce thickens.

11. Serve topped with scallions and garnish with lime wedges.

PER SERVING Calories: 360; Fat: 11g; Carbohydrates: 62g; Phosphorus: 120mg; Potassium: 193mg; Sodium: 166mg; Protein: 4g

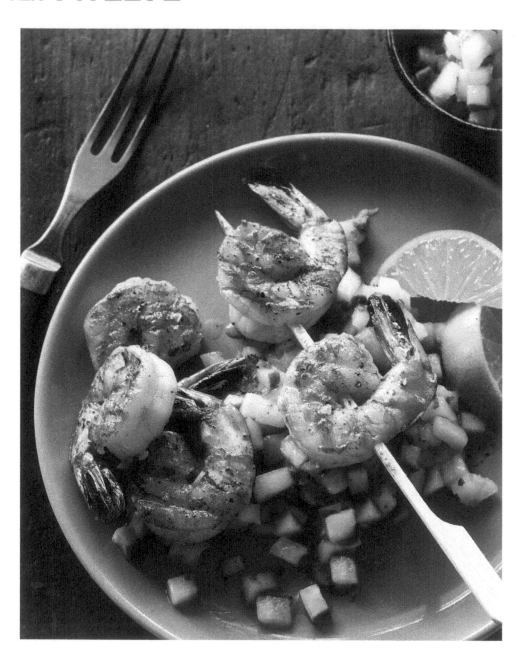

CHAPTER TWELVE

FISH AND SEAFOOD ENTRÉES

GRILLED SHRIMP WITH CUCUMBER LIME SALSA

Serves 4 / Prep time: 15 minutes / Cook time: 10 minutes

This dish is a visually pleasing creation composed of lime-infused mango cucumber salsa topped with grilled shrimp. You can create more visual impact with chopped bell pepper and a tablespoon of chopped cilantro. Remember to boil the red bell pepper to leach out some of the harmful minerals.

2 tablespoons olive oil
6 ounces large shrimp (16 to 20 count), peeled and deveined, tails left on
1 teaspoon minced garlic
½ cup chopped English cucumber
½ cup chopped mango
Zest of 1 lime
Juice of 1 lime
Freshly ground black pepper
Lime wedges for garnish

1. Soak 4 wooden skewers in water for 30 minutes.

2. Preheat the barbecue to medium-high heat.

3. In a large bowl, toss together the olive oil, shrimp, and garlic.

4. Thread the shrimp onto the skewers, about 4 shrimp per skewer.

5. In a small bowl, stir together the cucumber, mango, lime zest, and lime juice, and season the salsa lightly with pepper. Set aside.

6. Grill the shrimp for about 10 minutes, turning once or until the shrimp is opaque and cooked through.

7. Season the shrimp lightly with pepper.

8. Serve the shrimp on the cucumber salsa with lime wedges on the side.

PER SERVING Calories: 120; Fat: 8g; Carbohydrates: 4g; Phosphorus: 91mg; Potassium: 129mg; Sodium: 60mg; Protein: 9g

SHRIMP SCAMPI LINGUINE

Serves 4 / Prep time: 15 minutes / Cook time: 15 minutes

Shrimp may be small in size, but they are big in nutritional value. You do not need many shrimp in this recipe to create a flavor impact, and chopping them into smaller pieces will further distribute the flavor. Shrimp are low in calories and fat, rich in protein, and, like all seafood, high in heart-healthy omega-3 fatty acids.

4 ounces uncooked linguine

1 teaspoon olive oil

2 teaspoons minced garlic

4 ounces shrimp, peeled, deveined, and chopped

½ cup dry white wine

Juice of 1 lemon

1 tablespoon chopped fresh basil

½ cup heavy (whipping) cream

Freshly ground black pepper

1. Cook the linguine according to the package instructions; drain and set aside.

2. In a large skillet over medium heat, heat the olive oil.

3. Sauté the garlic and shrimp for about 6 minutes or until the shrimp is opaque and just cooked through.

4. Add the wine, lemon juice, and basil, and cook for 5 minutes.

5. Stir in the cream and simmer for 2 minutes more.

6. Add the linguine to the skillet and toss to coat.

7. Divide the pasta onto 4 plates to serve.

PER SERVING Calories: 219; Fat: 7g; Carbohydrates: 21g; Phosphorus: 119mg; Potassium: 155mg; Sodium: 42mg; Protein: 12g

CRAB CAKES WITH LIME SALSA

Serves 4 / Prep time: 20 minutes, plus 1 hour chilling time / Cook time: 20 minutes

Crab cakes are famous in many areas in the United States, such as Maryland and Seattle. This plump, sweet, and filling crab cake is both delicious and super easy to prepare. Crab meat is nutritious, too—low in calories and fat, and high in protein and heart-healthy omega-3 fatty acids. The salsa adds an unexpected citrus flare to the dish.

FOR THE SALSA

½ English cucumber, diced

1 lime, chopped

½ cup boiled and chopped red bell pepper

1 teaspoon chopped fresh cilantro

Freshly ground black pepper

FOR THE CRAB CAKES

8 ounces queen crab meat

¼ cup bread crumbs

1 small egg

¼ cup boiled and chopped red bell pepper

1 scallion, both green and white parts, minced

1 tablespoon chopped fresh parsley

Splash hot sauce

Olive oil spray, for the pan

TO MAKE THE SALSA

1. In a small bowl, stir together the cucumber, lime, red pepper, and cilantro.

2. Season with pepper; set aside.

TO MAKE THE CRAB CAKES

1. In a medium bowl, mix together the crab, bread crumbs, egg, red pepper, scallion, parsley, and hot sauce until it holds together. Add more bread crumbs, if necessary.

2. Form the crab mixture into 4 patties and place them on a plate.

3. Refrigerate the crab cakes for 1 hour to firm them.

4. Spray a large skillet generously with olive oil spray and place it over medium-high heat.

5. Cook the crab cakes in batches, turning, for about 5 minutes per side or until golden brown.

6. Serve the crab cakes with the salsa.

PER SERVING Calories: 115; Fat: 2g; Carbohydrates: 7g; Phosphorus: 110mg; Potassium: 200mg; Sodium: 421mg; Protein: 16g

SEAFOOD CASSEROLE

Serves 6 / Prep time: 20 minutes / Cook time: 45 minutes

If you like jambalaya, you will find the flavors and ingredient combination in this recipe familiar, but the process to make it is much simpler. Simply mix all the ingredients together and pop the dish in the oven until it is hot and bubbly. The hot sauce adds a fiery kick but can be easily omitted for a milder version of the dish.

2 cups eggplant, peeled and diced into 1-inch pieces
Butter, for greasing the baking dish
1 tablespoon olive oil
½ small sweet onion, chopped
1 teaspoon minced garlic
1 celery stalk, chopped
½ red bell pepper, boiled and chopped
3 tablespoons freshly squeezed lemon juice
1 teaspoon hot sauce
¼ teaspoon Creole Seasoning Mix (see page 93)
½ cup white rice, uncooked
1 large egg
4 ounces cooked shrimp
6 ounces queen crab meat

1. Preheat the oven to 350°F.
2. In a small saucepan filled with water over medium-high heat, boil the eggplant for 5 minutes. Drain and set aside in a large bowl.
3. Grease a 9-by-13-inch baking dish with butter and set aside.
4. In a large skillet over medium heat, heat the olive oil.
5. Sauté the onion, garlic, celery, and bell pepper for about 4 minutes or until they are tender.
6. Add the sautéed vegetables to the eggplant, along with the lemon juice, hot sauce, Creole seasoning, rice, and egg.
7. Stir to combine.

8. Fold in the shrimp and crab meat.

9. Spoon the casserole mixture into the casserole dish, patting down the top.

10. Bake for 25 to 30 minutes or until the casserole is heated through and the rice is tender.

11. Serve warm.

PER SERVING Calories: 118; Fat: 4g; Carbohydrates: 9g; Phosphorus: 102mg; Potassium: 199mg; Sodium: 235mg; Protein: 12g

SWEET GLAZED SALMON

Serves 4 / Prep time: 10 minutes / Cook time: 10 minutes

Honey is naturally acidic, so the simple rub used for this salmon creates tender flesh and a lovely golden crust. Different types of honey will impart unique flavors to the fish, such as a floral accent from clover honey or a more robust taste from buckwheat honey. The trick to a perfect coating is to pat the fish completely dry before applying the honey.

2 tablespoons honey

1 teaspoon lemon zest

½ teaspoon freshly ground black pepper

4 (3-ounce) salmon fillets

1 tablespoon olive oil

½ scallion, white and green parts, chopped

1. In a small bowl, stir together the honey, lemon zest, and pepper.
2. Wash the salmon and pat dry with paper towels.
3. Rub the honey mixture all over each fillet.
4. In a large skillet over medium heat, heat the olive oil.
5. Add the salmon fillets and cook the salmon for about 10 minutes, turning once, or until it is lightly browned and just cooked through.
6. Serve topped with chopped scallion.

Dialysis modification: *You can increase the amount of protein in this dish by eating 4 ounces of salmon instead of 3 ounces.*

PER SERVING Calories: 240; Fat: 15g; Carbohydrates: 9g; Phosphorus: 205mg; Potassium: 317mg; Sodium: 51mg; Protein: 17g

HERB-CRUSTED BAKED HADDOCK

Serves 4 / Prep time: 10 minutes / Cook time: 20 minutes

Buying fresh fish can be intimidating because determining quality can be difficult, but remember to examine the product closely. Fresh fish should have no strong fishy smell, the scales should be shiny, and the edges of the fillets should not be curled up or dry. This healthy, crispy haddock with the addition of fresh herbs and a touch of lemon zest is super quick to prepare and a perfect alternative to frozen, boxed fish.

½ cup bread crumbs

3 tablespoons chopped fresh parsley

1 tablespoon lemon zest

1 teaspoon chopped fresh thyme

¼ teaspoon freshly ground black pepper

1 tablespoon melted unsalted butter

12-ounces haddock fillets, deboned and skinned

1. Preheat the oven to 350°F.

2. In a small bowl, stir together the bread crumbs, parsley, lemon zest, thyme, and pepper until well combined.

3. Add the melted butter and toss until the mixture resembles coarse crumbs.

4. Place the haddock on a baking sheet and spoon the bread crumb mixture on top, pressing down firmly.

5. Bake the haddock in the oven for about 20 minutes or until the fish is just cooked through and flakes off in chunks when pressed.

Dialysis modification: *The haddock portion can be reduced to 2 ounces if you need to decrease the potassium and phosphorus. This will also reduce the protein.*

PER SERVING Calories: 143; Fat: 4g; Carbohydrates: 10g; Phosphorus: 216mg; Potassium: 285mg; Sodium: 281mg; Protein: 16g

SHORE LUNCH–STYLE SOLE

Serves 4 / Prep time: 20 minutes / Cook time: 10 minutes

This preparation for fish is common for fresh-caught trout because fisherman can easily carry plastic zipped bags of flour and a small container of oil with them on their boats. The flour-dusted fish will crisp up perfectly in hot oil. Sole is a more delicate fish than trout, so it takes a little less time in the skillet.

¼ cup all-purpose flour
¼ teaspoon freshly ground black pepper
12 ounces sole fillets, deboned and skinned
2 tablespoons olive oil
1 scallion, both green and white parts, chopped
Lemon wedges, for garnish

1. In a large plastic freezer bag, shake together the flour and pepper to combine.

2. Add the fish fillets to the flour and shake to coat.

3. In a large skillet over medium-high heat, heat the olive oil.

4. When the oil is hot, add the fish fillets and fry for about 10 minutes, turning once, or until they are golden and cooked through.

5. Remove the fish from the oil onto paper towels to drain.

6. Serve topped with chopped scallions and a squeeze of lemon.

Dialysis modification: *Most fish is high in phosphorus and potassium, so swapping out the sole for another fish might drop the levels a little. Balancing a meal with a little more phosphorus with lower-phosphorus meals the rest of the day is also a good strategy.*

PER SERVING Calories: 148; Fat: 8g; Carbohydrates: 6g; Phosphorus: 223mg; Potassium: 148mg; Sodium: 242mg; Protein: 11g

BAKED COD WITH CUCUMBER-DILL SALSA

Serves 4 / Prep time: 20 minutes / Cook time: 10 minutes

Baking is a quick and effective method to cook most types of fish, including cod. Drizzling the cod with olive oil and drenching the fillets in fresh lemon juice ensure the flesh remains moist when exposing it to the dry oven heat. Cover the fish with foil if you want a result that's even moister.

FOR THE CUCUMBER SALSA

½ English cucumber, chopped

2 tablespoons chopped fresh dill

Juice of 1 lime

Zest of 1 lime

¼ cup boiled and minced red bell pepper

½ teaspoon granulated sugar

FOR THE FISH

12 ounces cod fillets, deboned and cut into 4 servings

Juice of 1 lemon

½ teaspoon freshly ground black pepper

1 teaspoon olive oil

TO MAKE THE CUCUMBER SALSA

In a small bowl, mix together the cucumber, dill, lime juice, lime zest, red pepper, and sugar; set aside. ▶

TO MAKE THE FISH

1. Preheat the oven to 350°F.

2. Place the fish on a pie plate and squeeze the lemon juice evenly over the fillets.

3. Sprinkle with pepper and drizzle the olive oil evenly over the fillets.

4. Bake the fish for about 6 minutes or until it flakes easily with a fork.

5. Transfer the fish to 4 plates and serve topped with cucumber salsa.

Dialysis modification: *To reduce the amount of potassium, try this baked fish with a sprinkling of fresh dill and a little lime zest instead of the salsa.*

PER SERVING   Calories: 110; Fat: 2g; Carbohydrates: 3g; Phosphorus: 120mg; Potassium: 275mg; Sodium: 67mg; Protein: 20g

CILANTRO-LIME FLOUNDER

Serves 4 / Prep time: 20 minutes / Cook time: 5 minutes

If you need to boost your protein intake, flounder is a wonderful choice because it is a high-quality, complete protein containing all essential amino acids. Flounder is a delicate fish that can dry out with the wrong cooking method, but the protective coating of mayonnaise in this preparation creates a moist and flaky result.

¼ cup Homemade Mayonnaise (see page 71)
Juice of 1 lime
Zest of 1 lime
½ cup chopped fresh cilantro
4 (3-ounce) flounder fillets
Freshly ground black pepper

1. Preheat the oven to 400°F.

2. In a small bowl, stir together the mayonnaise, lime juice, lime zest, and cilantro.

3. Place 4 pieces of foil, about 8 by 8 inches square, on a clean work surface.

4. Place a flounder fillet in the center of each square.

5. Top the fillets evenly with the mayonnaise mixture.

6. Season the flounder with pepper.

7. Fold the sides of the foil over the fish, creating a snug packet, and place the foil packets on a baking sheet.

8. Bake the fish 4 to 5 minutes.

9. Unfold the packets and serve.

PER SERVING Calories: 92; Fat: 4g; Carbohydrates: 2g; Phosphorus: 208mg; Potassium: 137mg; Sodium: 267mg; Protein: 12g

HERB PESTO TUNA

Serves 4 / Prep time: 10 minutes / Cook time: 10 minutes

Tuna is a great addition to your diet for heart health. As with other oily fish, tuna is full of omega-3 fatty acids, which lower triglycerides, a form of fat found in the blood. Omega 3s may also slow down the growth of plaque in arteries and reduce inflammation throughout the body. How you prepare the fish is important, too: Broiling, steaming, or grilling are the most heart-healthy choices.

4 (3-ounce) yellowfin tuna fillets
1 teaspoon olive oil
Freshly ground black pepper
¼ cup Herb Pesto (see page 73)
1 lemon, cut into 8 thin slices

1. Heat the barbecue to medium-high.

2. Drizzle the fish with the olive oil and season each fillet with pepper.

3. Cook the fish on the barbecue for 4 minutes.

4. Turn the fish over and top each piece with the herb pesto and lemon slices.

5. Grill for 5 to 6 minutes more or until the tuna is cooked to medium-well.

Dialysis modification: *The pesto adds about 15 mg of potassium to this recipe. The tuna is the reason the recipe is high in potassium. Try this recipe with other fish such as haddock or cod, but broil the fish instead of putting it on the barbecue.*

PER SERVING   Calories: 103; Fat: 2g; Carbohydrates: 0g; Phosphorus: 236mg; Potassium: 374mg; Sodium: 38mg; Protein: 21g

GRILLED CALAMARI WITH LEMON AND HERBS

Serves 4 / Prep time: 10 minutes, plus 1 hour for marinating / Cook time: 3 minutes

When shopping for calamari in your local grocery store, look for squid on the label or at the fish counter because calamari is the Italian word for this tasty sea creature. If you cannot find fresh squid, purchase it frozen and thaw it completely before marinating it in the olive oil mixture. Calamari can get overcooked very quickly and become rubbery, so watch your cooking time closely and eat soon after removing the squid from the heat.

2 tablespoons olive oil
2 tablespoons freshly squeezed lemon juice
1 tablespoon chopped fresh parsley
1 tablespoon chopped fresh oregano
2 teaspoons minced garlic
Pinch sea salt
Pinch freshly ground black pepper
½ pound cleaned calamari
Lemon wedges, for garnish

1. In large bowl, stir together the olive oil, lemon juice, parsley, oregano, garlic, salt, and pepper.

2. Add the calamari to the bowl and stir to coat.

3. Cover the bowl and refrigerate the calamari for 1 hour to marinate.

4. Preheat the barbecue to medium-high.

5. Grill the calamari, turning once, until firm and opaque, about 3 minutes total.

6. Serve with lemon wedges.

PER SERVING Calories: 81; Fat: 7g; Carbohydrates: 2g; Phosphorus: 128mg; Potassium: 160mg; Sodium: 67mg; Protein: 3g

CHAPTER THIRTEEN

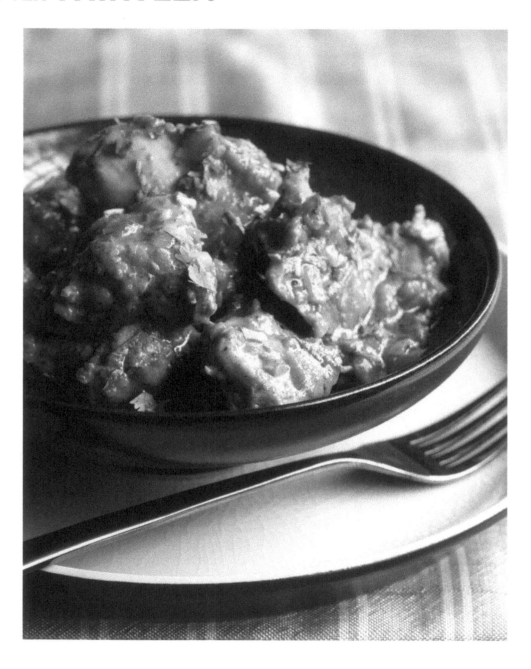

MEAT AND POULTRY ENTRÉES

LEMON-HERB CHICKEN

Serves 4 / Prep time: 20 minutes / Cook time: 15 minutes

Lemons, part of the citrus family, are on the American Diabetes Association's list of diabetes superfoods because they are high in soluble fiber and vitamin C. Soluble fiber helps stabilize blood-sugar levels, which helps people with diabetes better manage their condition. Lemons are a great addition to recipes, providing flavor to food without the need for salt or sugar.

12 ounces boneless, skinless chicken breast, cut into 8 strips
1 small egg white
2 tablespoons water, divided
½ cup bread crumbs
¼ cup unsalted butter, divided
Juice of 1 lemon
Zest of 1 lemon
1 tablespoon fresh chopped basil
1 teaspoon fresh chopped thyme
Lemon slices, for garnish

1. Place the chicken strips between 2 sheets of plastic wrap and pound each flat with a mallet or rolling pin.

2. In a medium bowl, whisk together the egg and 1 tablespoon water.

3. Put the bread crumbs in another medium bowl.

4. Dredge the chicken strips, one at a time, in the egg, then the bread crumbs, and set the breaded strips aside on a plate.

5. In a large skillet over medium heat, melt 2 tablespoons of the butter.

6. Cook the strips in the butter for about 3 minutes, turning once, or until they are golden and cooked through.

7. Transfer the chicken to a plate.

8. Add the lemon juice, lemon zest, basil, thyme, and remaining 1 tablespoon water to the skillet and stir until the mixture simmers.

9. Remove the sauce from the heat and stir in the remaining 2 tablespoons butter.

10. Serve the chicken with the lemon sauce drizzled over the top and garnished with lemon slices.

PER SERVING Calories: 255; Fat: 14g; Carbohydrates: 11g; Phosphorus: 180mg; Potassium: 321mg; Sodium: 261mg; Protein: 20g

ASIAN CHICKEN SATAY

Serves 6 / Prep time: 15 minutes, plus 1 hour for marinating / Cook time: 10 minutes

This dish makes a nice light meal with rice pilaf and a huge, fresh green salad. Soak the wooden skewers in water for at least 30 minutes before threading on the chicken, to ensure the skewers will not catch fire on the barbecue. If you do not have a barbecue, broil the chicken for 5 minutes per side in the oven.

Juice of 2 limes
2 tablespoons brown sugar
1 tablespoon minced garlic
2 teaspoons ground cumin
12 ounces boneless, skinless chicken breast, cut into 12 strips

1. In a large bowl, stir together the lime juice, brown sugar, garlic, and cumin.

2. Add the chicken strips to the bowl and marinate in the refrigerator for 1 hour.

3. Heat the barbecue to medium-high.

4. Remove the chicken from the marinade and thread each strip onto wooden skewers that have been soaked in water.

5. Grill the chicken for about 4 minutes per side or until the meat is cooked through but still juicy.

PER SERVING Calories: 78; Fat: 2g; Carbohydrates: 4g; Phosphorus: 116mg; Potassium: 208mg; Sodium: 100mg; Protein: 12g

CHICKEN STIR-FRY

Serves 5 / Prep time: 20 minutes / Cook time: 15 minutes

Staggering the addition of vegetables and meat when stir-frying is essential to avoid overcooked, limp snow peas or hard, undercooked cauliflower. Heartier vegetables should always be added first to give them more time over the heat. When chicken is a part of your stir-fry, put it in the skillet first to make sure it gets cooked thoroughly.

3 tablespoons pineapple juice

1 tablespoon balsamic vinegar

1 teaspoon grated fresh ginger

1 teaspoon minced garlic

2 teaspoons cornstarch

2 tablespoons olive oil

12 ounces boneless, skinless chicken breast, cut into 1-inch chunks

½ cup cauliflower florets

½ cup carrots, cut into thin disks

½ cup green beans

3 cups cooked white rice

1. In a small bowl, stir together the pineapple juice, balsamic vinegar, garlic, ginger, and cornstarch; set aside.

2. In a large skillet or wok over medium-high heat, heat the olive oil.

3. Sauté the chicken for about 6 minutes or until it is just cooked through. Remove the cooked chicken to a plate.

4. Add the cauliflower, carrots, and green beans to the skillet and stir-fry for about 4 minutes or until the vegetables are crisp and tender.

5. Return the chicken to the skillet and toss to combine. ▶

6. Push the chicken and vegetables over to the side of the skillet and pour the sauce into the empty spot.

7. Cook for about 2 minutes, stirring, or until the sauce is thickened.

8. Stir the vegetables and chicken back into the sauce to coat.

9. Serve over rice.

PER SERVING Calories: 161; Fat: 5g; Carbohydrates: 18g; Phosphorus: 96mg; Potassium: 208mg; Sodium: 90mg; Protein: 11g

INDIAN CHICKEN CURRY

Serves 6 / Prep time: 20 minutes / Cook time: 40 minutes

Chicken thighs are juicy, flavorful, and braise beautifully. It can be difficult to debone thighs well, so try to purchase them already deboned to save time and effort. If you do debone them yourself, save the thigh bones in the fridge or freezer to make a homemade chicken stock at a later time.

3 tablespoons olive oil, divided

6 boneless, skinless chicken thighs

1 small sweet onion

2 teaspoons minced garlic

1 teaspoon grated fresh ginger

1 tablespoon Hot Curry Powder (see page 87)

¾ cup water

¼ cup coconut milk

2 tablespoons chopped fresh cilantro

1. In a large skillet over a medium-high heat, heat 2 tablespoons of the oil.

2. Add the chicken and cook for about 10 minutes or until the thighs are browned all over.

3. With tongs, remove the chicken to a plate and set aside.

4. Add the remaining 1 tablespoon of oil to the skillet and sauté the onion, garlic, and ginger for about 3 minutes or until they are softened.

5. Stir in the curry powder, water, and coconut milk.

6. Return the chicken to the skillet and bring the liquid to a boil.

7. Reduce the heat to low, cover the skillet, and simmer for about 25 minutes or until the chicken is tender and the sauce is thick.

8. Serve topped with cilantro.

PER SERVING Calories: 241; Fat: 14g; Carbohydrates: 2g; Phosphorus: 145mg; Potassium: 230mg; Sodium: 76mg; Protein: 26g

PERSIAN CHICKEN

Serves 5 / Prep time: 10 minutes, plus 2 hours for marinating / Cook time: 20 minutes

This marinade can be used with pork or chicken thighs because the spices and lemon flavor complement these meats beautifully. For better infusion of the marinade, prick the pork or chicken all over with a fork before marinating. This will allow the flavors to penetrate below the surface.

½ small sweet onion, chopped
¼ cup freshly squeezed lemon juice
1 tablespoon dried oregano
1 teaspoon minced garlic
1 teaspoon sweet paprika
½ teaspoon ground cumin
½ cup olive oil
5 boneless, skinless chicken thighs

1. Put the onion, lemon juice, oregano, garlic, paprika, and cumin in a blender or food processor.
2. Pulse a few times to mix the ingredients.
3. With the motor running, add the olive oil until the mixture is smooth.
4. Place the chicken thighs in a large sealable freezer bag and pour the marinade into the bag.
5. Seal the bag and place it in the refrigerator, turning the bag twice, for 2 hours.
6. Remove the thighs from the marinade and discard the extra marinade.
7. Preheat the barbecue to medium.
8. Grill the chicken for about 20 minutes, turning once, or until the internal temperature is 165°F.

PER SERVING Calories: 321; Fat: 21g; Carbohydrates: 3g; Phosphorus: 131mg; Potassium: 220mg; Sodium: 86mg; Protein: 22g

PESTO PORK CHOPS

Serves 4 / Prep time: 20 minutes / Cook time: 20 minutes

Pork, sometimes called "the other white meat," can be compared to chicken in terms of nutrition benefits. Pork is higher in protein and lower in cholesterol than chicken, and it has about the same number of calories per serving. Cooking pork chops in a coating of bread crumbs seals in the flavor and tasty juices, so the meat will never be dry.

4 (3-ounce) pork top-loin chops, boneless, fat trimmed
8 teaspoons Herb Pesto (page 73)
½ cup bread crumbs
1 tablespoon olive oil

1. Preheat the oven to 450°F.
2. Line a baking sheet with foil; set aside.
3. Rub 1 teaspoon of pesto evenly over both sides of each pork chop.
4. Lightly dredge each pork chop in the bread crumbs.
5. In a large skillet over medium-high heat, heat the oil.
6. Brown the pork chops on each side for about 5 minutes.
7. Place the pork chops on the baking sheet.
8. Bake for about 10 minutes or until the pork reaches 145°F in the center.

PER SERVING Calories: 210; Fat: 7g; Carbohydrates: 10g; Phosphorus: 179mg; Potassium: 220mg; Sodium: 148mg; Protein: 24g

PORK SOUVLAKI

Serves 8 / Prep time: 20 minutes, plus 2 hours for marinating / Cook time: 12 minutes

Souvlaki is a Greek street food that typically features lamb instead of pork. The appeal of souvlaki and other Greek street food, such as gyros, is the freshness of the ingredients and flavorful marinades. If you need a more substantial meal, slide the cooked pork into a warmed pita bread pocket and top with shredded cucumber and lettuce.

3 tablespoons olive oil
2 tablespoons lemon juice
1 teaspoon minced garlic
1 tablespoon chopped fresh oregano
¼ teaspoon freshly ground black pepper
1 pound pork leg, cut in 2-inch cubes

1. In a medium bowl, stir together the olive oil, lemon juice, garlic, oregano, and pepper.
2. Add the pork cubes and toss to coat.
3. Place the bowl in the refrigerator, covered, for 2 hours to marinate.
4. Thread the pork chunks onto 8 metal skewers or wood skewers that have been soaked in water.
5. Preheat the barbecue to medium-high heat.
6. Grill the pork skewers for about 12 minutes, turning once, until just cooked through but still juicy.

PER SERVING Calories: 95; Fat: 4g; Carbohydrates: 0g; Phosphorus: 125mg; Potassium: 230mg; Sodium: 29mg; Protein: 13g

CHILI-ROASTED PORK LEG

Serves 6 / Prep time: 10 minutes, plus 3 hours for marinating / Cook time: 50 minutes

Pork leg is not a label you typically see at your local supermarket meat counter, but you might know it by its more common name: fresh ham. This cut of pork is from the hind leg of a pig and can be purchased bone-in or boneless, depending on your needs. You might have to order a pork leg from the local butcher because most are cured into hams, but the extra effort is worth the end result.

2 teaspoons chili powder

2 teaspoons ground allspice

1½ teaspoons ground cumin

1 teaspoon garlic powder

1 teaspoon ground cinnamon

½ teaspoon freshly ground black pepper

Pinch cayenne pepper

1 pound boneless pork leg roast

2 tablespoons olive oil

1. In a small bowl, mix together the chili powder, allspice, cumin, garlic powder, cinnamon, black pepper, and cayenne pepper.

2. Rub the spice mixture generously all over the pork leg.

3. Place the pork loin in the refrigerator to marinate for 3 hours.

4. Preheat the oven to 350°F.

5. In a large skillet over medium-high heat, heat the olive oil.

6. Sear the pork loin on all sides and transfer it to a baking dish.

7. Roast, uncovered, for about 40 minutes or until the internal temperature reaches 160°F.

8. Remove the pork from the oven and let it rest for 10 minutes.

9. Cut into thin slices to serve.

PER SERVING Calories: 98; Fat: 4g; Carbohydrates: 1g; Phosphorus: 130mg; Potassium: 240mg; Sodium: 29mg; Protein: 13g

OPEN-FACED BEEF STIR-UP

Serves 6 / Prep time: 10 minutes / Cook time: 10 minutes

This messy sandwich is easy, fast, and surprisingly tasty. You could also add the top bun and shredded lettuce for a more traditional presentation, but don't be afraid to get messy! Extra-lean turkey or chicken could be substituted for beef in this recipe if you have those ingredients on hand instead.

½ pound 95% lean ground beef
½ cup chopped sweet onion
½ cup shredded cabbage
¼ cup Herb Pesto (see page 73)
6 hamburger buns, bottom halves only

1. In a large skillet over medium heat, sauté the beef and onion for about 6 minutes or until the beef is cooked.

2. Add the cabbage and sauté for 3 additional minutes.

3. Stir in the pesto and heat for 1 minute.

4. Divide the beef mixture into 6 portions and serve each on the bottom half of a hamburger bun, open-face.

PER SERVING   Calories: 120; Fat: 3g; Carbohydrates: 13g; Phosphorus: 106mg; Potassium: 198mg; Sodium: 134mg; Protein: 11g

SWEET AND SOUR MEAT LOAF

Serves 8 / Prep time: 10 minutes / Cook time: 50 minutes

Meat loaf is inexpensive to make and a versatile meal that can be customized any way you like, depending on your palate and budget. If you are feeling ambitious, make two meat loaves and freeze the second one for another meal. Or, use slices of cold meat loaf for sandwiches. This recipe would work nicely with ground chicken or pork as well.

1 pound 95% lean ground beef
½ cup bread crumbs
½ cup chopped sweet onion
1 large egg
2 tablespoons chopped fresh basil
1 teaspoon chopped fresh thyme
1 teaspoon chopped fresh parsley
¼ teaspoon freshly ground black pepper
1 tablespoon brown sugar
1 teaspoon white vinegar
¼ teaspoon garlic powder

1. Preheat the oven to 350°F.
2. Mix together the beef, bread crumbs, onion, egg, basil, thyme, parsley, and pepper until well combined.
3. Press the meat mixture into a 9-by-5-inch loaf pan.
4. In a small bowl, stir together the brown sugar, vinegar, and garlic powder.
5. Spread the brown sugar mixture evenly over the meat.
6. Bake the meat loaf for about 50 minutes or until it is cooked through.
7. Let the meat loaf stand for 10 minutes and then pour out any accumulated grease.

PER SERVING Calories: 103; Fat: 3g; Carbohydrates: 7g; Phosphorus: 112mg; Potassium: 190mg; Sodium: 87mg; Protein: 11g

GRILLED STEAK WITH CUCUMBER-CILANTRO SALSA

Serves 4 / Prep time: 20 minutes / Cook time: 15 minutes

Beef tenderloin is considered the Cadillac of beef choices because it sits right beneath the ribs on the cow, a part of the animal that moves very little, making the cut very tender. It also has very little fat marbling, making it an excellent choice for people who love the flavor of steak but are limiting the amount of fat in their diet. For a consistent diameter and size, try to purchase the center cut of the tenderloin rather than the butt (thick end) or tail (thin end) portions.

FOR THE SALSA

1 cup chopped English cucumber
¼ cup boiled and diced red bell pepper
1 scallion, both green and white parts, chopped
2 tablespoons chopped fresh cilantro
Juice of 1 lime

FOR THE STEAK

4 (3-ounce) beef tenderloin steaks
Olive oil
Freshly ground black pepper

TO MAKE THE SALSA

In a medium bowl, combine the cucumber, bell pepper, scallion, cilantro, and lime juice; set aside.

TO MAKE THE STEAK

1. Preheat a barbecue to medium-high.

2. Take the steaks out of the refrigerator and let them come to room temperature.

3. Rub the steaks all over with olive oil and season with pepper.

4. Grill the steaks for about 5 minutes per side for medium-rare, or until desired doneness.

5. If you do not have a barbecue, broil the steaks in the oven for 6 minutes per side for medium-rare.

6. Let the steaks rest for 10 minutes.

7. Serve the steaks topped with the salsa.

PER SERVING Calories: 130; Fat: 6g; Carbohydrates: 1g; Phosphorus: 186mg; Potassium: 272mg; Sodium: 39mg; Protein: 19g

CLASSIC POT ROAST

Serves 8 / Prep time: 10 minutes / Cook time: 5 hours

Recipes for modern-day pot roast date back to 1881, although variations on this braised dish stretch back centuries. Pot roast is a Sunday-night staple in many homes because it can be prepared all in one pot for easy cleanup, and it can be left to cook all day. You can even place the browned meat into a slow cooker and let it cook on low for 8 hours for a delicious, no-fuss supper.

1 pound boneless beef chuck or rump roast
½ teaspoon freshly ground black pepper
1 tablespoon olive oil
½ small sweet onion, chopped
2 teaspoons minced garlic
1 teaspoon dried thyme
1 cup plus 3 tablespoons water
2 tablespoons cornstarch

1. Place a large stockpot over medium heat.

2. Season the roast with pepper.

3. Add the oil to the stockpot and brown the meat all over.

4. Remove the meat to a plate; set aside.

5. Sauté the onion and garlic in the stockpot for about 3 minutes or until they are softened.

6. Return the beef to the pot with any accumulated juices and add the thyme and 1 cup water.

7. Bring the liquid to a boil and then reduce the heat to low so that the liquid simmers.

8. Cover and simmer for about 4½ hours or until the beef is very tender.

9. In a small bowl, stir together the cornstarch and 3 tablespoons water to form a slurry.

10. Whisk the slurry into the liquid in the pot and cook for 15 minutes to thicken the sauce.

11. Serve the roast with the gravy.

PER SERVING Calories: 159; Fat: 10g; Carbohydrates: 2g; Phosphorus: 109mg; Potassium: 184mg; Sodium: 44mg; Protein: 14g

CHAPTER FOURTEEN

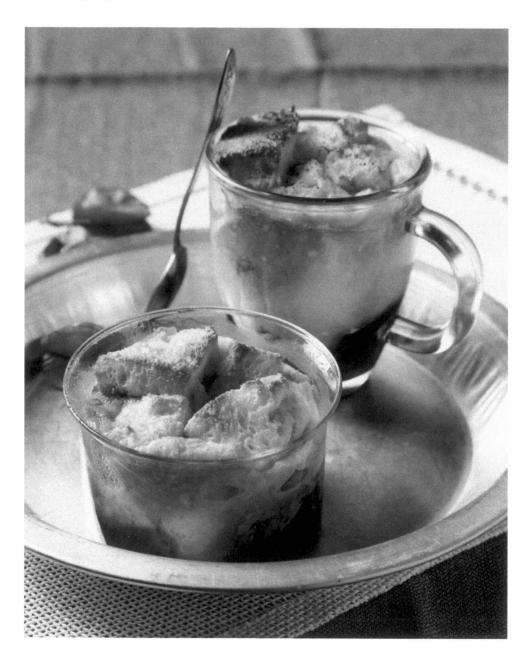

DESSERTS

TART APPLE GRANITA

Serves 4 / Prep time: 15 minutes, plus 4 hours freezing time

Granita has a pleasing texture from the large ice crystals that form when the liquid freezes. For a more intense apple flavor, you can juice fresh apples instead of using prepared juice from a can or bottle. Granny Smith, McIntosh, or Spartan apples are the best choices for a truly tart iced treat.

½ cup granulated sugar
½ cup water
2 cups unsweetened apple juice
¼ cup freshly squeezed lemon juice

1. In a small saucepan over medium-high heat, heat the sugar and water.
2. Bring the mixture to a boil and then reduce the heat to low and simmer for about 15 minutes or until the liquid has reduced by half.
3. Remove the pan from the heat and pour the liquid into a large shallow metal pan.
4. Let the liquid cool for about 30 minutes and then stir in the apple juice and lemon juice.
5. Place the pan in the freezer.
6. After 1 hour, run a fork through the liquid to break up any ice crystals that have formed. Scrape down the sides as well.
7. Place the pan back in the freezer and repeat the stirring and scraping every 20 minutes, creating slush.
8. Serve when the mixture is completely frozen and looks like crushed ice, after about 3 hours.

PER SERVING Calories: 157; Fat: 0g; Carbohydrates: 0g; Phosphorus: 10mg; Potassium: 141mg; Sodium: 5mg; Protein: 0g

LEMON-LIME SHERBET

Serves 8 / Prep time: 5 minutes, plus 3 hours chilling time / Cook time: 15 minutes

Sherbet is the creamier version of sorbet. A little cream or milk is added to what is essentially a sorbet mixture, and the result is a frozen dessert that's richer than sorbet but lighter than ice cream. This sherbet has heavy cream as its dairy component and is a nice, tart choice for a refreshing summertime dessert. Top a bowl of this sherbet with fresh mint sprigs and a sprinkle of toasted coconut for a special finish.

2 cups water

1 cup granulated sugar

3 tablespoons lemon zest, divided

½ cup freshly squeezed lemon juice

Zest of 1 lime

Juice of 1 lime

½ cup heavy (whipping) cream

1. Place a large saucepan over medium-high heat and add the water, sugar, and 2 tablespoons of the lemon zest.

2. Bring the mixture to a boil and then reduce the heat and simmer for 15 minutes.

3. Transfer the mixture to a large bowl and add the remaining 1 tablespoon lemon zest, the lemon juice, lime zest, and lime juice.

4. Chill the mixture in the fridge until completely cold, about 3 hours.

5. Whisk in the heavy cream and transfer the mixture to an ice cream maker.

6. Freeze according to the manufacturer's instructions.

PER SERVING Calories: 151; Fat: 6g; Carbohydrates: 26g; Phosphorus: 10mg; Potassium: 27mg; Sodium: 6mg; Protein: 0g

TROPICAL VANILLA SNOW CONE

Serves 4 / Prep time: 15 minutes, plus freezing time

The best way to serve this sweet, pale pink treat is in old-fashioned pointed paper cups to mimic the look of a real snow cone. If you want to save time creating the icy texture, pop the entire frozen-fruit mixture out of the dish and pulse it in a food processor until it resembles snow. This will only work if you are serving the dessert right away and you eat all of it in one sitting.

1 cup canned peaches
1 cup pineapple
1 cup frozen strawberries
6 tablespoons water
2 tablespoons granulated sugar
1 tablespoon vanilla extract

1. In a large saucepan, mix together the peaches, pineapple, strawberries, water, and sugar over medium-high heat and bring to a boil.

2. Reduce the heat to low and simmer the mixture, stirring occasionally, for 15 minutes.

3. Remove from the heat and let the mixture cool completely, for about 1 hour.

4. Stir in the vanilla and transfer the fruit mixture to a food processor or blender.

5. Purée until smooth, and pour the purée into a 9-by-13-inch glass baking dish.

6. Cover and place the dish in the freezer overnight.

7. When the fruit mixture is completely frozen, use a fork to scrape the sorbet until you have flaked flavored ice.

8. Scoop the ice flakes into 4 serving dishes.

PER SERVING   Calories: 92; Fat: 0g; Carbohydrates: 22g; Phosphorus: 17mg; Potassium: 145mg; Sodium: 4mg; Protein: 1g

PAVLOVA WITH PEACHES

Serves 8 / Prep time: 30 minutes / Cook time: 1 hour, plus cooling time

Pavlovas are a simple, baked meringue topped with fruit, chocolate, or sauces. Meringue is not difficult to make, but some simple tricks will ensure success. Separate the eggs when they are cold, so the yolks are less likely to break. Even the slightest hint of yolk in the whites can impede the beating process. Crack the eggs individually over a glass and then transfer the white into a bowl, so only one egg white will be ruined if the yolk breaks.

4 large egg whites, at room temperature

½ teaspoon cream of tartar

1 cup superfine sugar

½ teaspoon pure vanilla extract

2 cups drained canned peaches in juice

1. Preheat the oven to 225°F.

2. Line a baking sheet with parchment paper; set aside.

3. In a large bowl, beat the egg whites for about 1 minute or until soft peaks form.

4. Beat in the cream of tartar.

5. Add the sugar, 1 tablespoon at a time, until the egg whites are very stiff and glossy. Do not overbeat.

6. Beat in the vanilla.

7. Evenly spoon the meringue onto the baking sheet so that you have 8 rounds.

8. Use the back of the spoon to create an indentation in the middle of each round.

9. Bake the meringues for about 1 hour or until a light brown crust forms.

10. Turn off the oven and let the meringues stand, still in the oven, overnight.

11. Remove the meringues from the sheet and place them on serving plates.

12. Spoon the peaches, dividing evenly, into the centers of the meringues, and serve.

13. Store any unused meringues in a sealed container at room temperature for up to 1 week.

PER SERVING Calories: 132; Fat: 0g; Carbohydrates: 32g; Phosphorus: 7mg; Potassium: 95mg; Sodium: 30mg; Protein: 2g

BAKED PEACHES WITH CREAM CHEESE

Serves 4 / Prep time: 10 minutes / Cook time: 15 minutes

Canned peaches become an elegant, rich dessert when stuffed with sweet, crunchy cookie crumbles, tart cream cheese, and honey. Peaches packed in juice, water, or light syrup are the best choice for this recipe. Peaches are an excellent source of fiber and vitamins A and C.

1 cup plain cream cheese, at room temperature
½ cup crushed Meringue Cookies (see page 131)
¼ teaspoon ground cinnamon
Pinch ground nutmeg
8 canned peach halves, in juice
2 tablespoons honey

1. Preheat the oven to 350°F.
2. Line a baking sheet with parchment paper; set aside.
3. In a small bowl, stir together the cream cheese, meringue cookies, cinnamon, and nutmeg.
4. Spoon the cream cheese mixture evenly into the cavities in the peach halves.
5. Place the peaches on the baking sheet and bake for about 15 minutes or until the fruit is soft and the cheese is melted.
6. Remove the peaches from the baking sheet onto plates, 2 per person, and drizzle with honey before serving.

PER SERVING Calories: 260; Fat: 20g; Carbohydrates: 19g; Phosphorus: 74mg; Potassium: 198mg; Sodium: 216mg; Protein: 4g

SWEET CINNAMON CUSTARD

Serves 6 / Prep time: 20 minutes, plus 1 hour chilling time / Cook time: 1 hour

Baked custards are cool and creamy with a velvety smoothness. A moist cooking environment is essential to avoid curdling the custard mixture like scrambled eggs, so always remember the water-bath step. Try adding carob powder, fruit purée, coffee, and other flavoring extracts for unique variations of this basic custard recipe.

Unsalted butter, for greasing the ramekins
1½ cups plain rice milk
4 eggs
¼ cup granulated sugar
1 teaspoon pure vanilla extract
½ teaspoon ground cinnamon
Cinnamon sticks, for garnish (optional)

1. Preheat the oven to 325°F.
2. Lightly grease 6 (4-ounce) ramekins and place them in a baking dish; set aside.
3. In a large bowl, whisk together the rice milk, eggs, sugar, vanilla, and cinnamon until the mixture is very smooth.
4. Pour the mixture through a fine sieve into a pitcher.
5. Evenly divide the custard mixture among the ramekins.
6. Fill the baking dish with hot water, taking care not to get any water in the ramekins, until the water reaches halfway up the sides of the ramekins.
7. Bake for about 1 hour or until the custards are set and a knife inserted in the center of one of the custards comes out clean.
8. Remove the custards from the oven and take the ramekins out of the water.
9. Cool on wire racks for 1 hour and then transfer the custards to the refrigerator to chill for an additional hour.
10. Garnish each custard with a cinnamon stick, if desired.

PER SERVING   Calories: 110; Fat: 4g; Carbohydrates: 14g; Phosphorus: 100mg; Potassium: 64mg; Sodium: 71mg; Protein: 4g

RASPBERRY BRÛLÉE

Serves 4 / Prep time: 15 minutes / Cook time: 1 minute

This dessert is not the crème brûlée you might have eaten in high-end restaurants. You will not need to fiddle with water baths to create the smooth, tart base of this dessert; it is unbaked and simple. The burned sugar or brûlée happens in the oven, but if you want to create the crackly, caramelized sugar crust like a professional chef, use a handheld kitchen torch on each ramekin.

½ cup light sour cream
½ cup plain cream cheese, at room temperature
¼ cup brown sugar, divided
¼ teaspoon ground cinnamon
1 cup fresh raspberries

1. Preheat the oven to broil.
2. In a small bowl, beat together the sour cream, cream cheese, 2 tablespoons brown sugar, and cinnamon for about 4 minutes or until the mixture is very smooth and fluffy.
3. Evenly divide the raspberries among 4 (4-ounce) ramekins.
4. Spoon the cream cheese mixture over the berries and smooth the tops.
5. Store the ramekins in the refrigerator, covered, until you are ready to serve the dessert.
6. Sprinkle ½ tablespoon brown sugar evenly over each ramekin.
7. Place the ramekins on a baking sheet and broil 4 inches from the heating element until the sugar is caramelized and golden brown.
8. Remove from the oven. Let the brûlées sit 1 minute, and serve.

PER SERVING Calories: 188; Fat: 13g; Carbohydrates: 16g; Phosphorus: 60mg; Potassium: 158mg; Sodium: 132mg; Protein: 3g

VANILLA-INFUSED COUSCOUS PUDDING

Serves 6 / Prep time: 20 minutes / Cook time: 20 minutes

Couscous replaces rice in this dish, creating a slightly different taste and a unique texture. The vanilla bean adds superior flavor to the pudding, but you can substitute extract if you do not have beans. Look for whole vanilla beans in the baking section of your local grocery store.

1½ cups plain rice milk
½ cup water
1 vanilla bean, split
½ cup honey
¼ teaspoon ground cinnamon
1 cup couscous

1. In a large saucepan, mix together the rice milk, water, and vanilla bean in large saucepan over medium heat.

2. Bring the milk to a gentle simmer, reduce the heat to low, and let the milk simmer for 10 minutes to allow the vanilla flavor to infuse into the milk.

3. Remove the saucepan from the heat.

4. Take out the vanilla bean and, using the tip of a paring knife, scrape the seeds from the pod into the warm milk.

5. Stir in the honey and cinnamon.

6. Stir in the couscous, cover the pan, and let it stand for 10 minutes.

7. With a fork, fluff the couscous before serving.

PER SERVING Calories: 334; Fat: 1g; Carbohydrates: 77g; Phosphorus: 119mg; Potassium: 118mg; Sodium: 41mg; Protein: 6g

HONEY BREAD PUDDING

Serves 6 / Prep time: 15 minutes, plus 3 hours soaking time / Cook time: 40 minutes

This version of bread pudding is similar to tender French toast sliced into large pieces. The soft bread is infused with the egg and milk mixture, creating a velvety custard and a caramelized golden crust. Try topping this dessert with an extra drizzle of honey and fresh whipped cream.

Unsalted butter, for greasing the baking dish
1½ cups plain rice milk
2 eggs
2 large egg whites
¼ cup honey
1 teaspoon pure vanilla extract
6 cups cubed white bread

1. Lightly grease an 8-by-8-inch baking dish with butter; set aside.
2. In a medium bowl, whisk together the rice milk, eggs, egg whites, honey, and vanilla.
3. Add the bread cubes and stir until the bread is coated.
4. Transfer the mixture to the baking dish and cover with plastic wrap.
5. Store the dish in the refrigerator at least 3 hours.
6. Preheat the oven to 325°F.
7. Remove the plastic wrap from the baking dish and bake the pudding for 35 to 40 minutes or until golden brown and a knife inserted in the center comes out clean.
8. Serve warm.

PER SERVING Calories: 167; Fat: 3g; Carbohydrates: 30g; Phosphorus: 95mg; Potassium: 93mg; Sodium: 189mg; Protein: 6g

RHUBARB CRUMBLE

Serves 6 / Prep time: 15 minutes / Cook time: 30 minutes

Fruit crumble belongs in a delicious dessert category that includes crisps, brown Betty, and cobblers. Crumbles usually do not contain nuts or oats, so the topping seems more like a butter cookie than a crust. Make this crumble with any kind of fruit, depending on the season and your personal preference.

Unsalted butter, for greasing the baking dish
1 cup all-purpose flour
½ cup brown sugar
½ teaspoon ground cinnamon
½ cup unsalted butter, at room temperature
1 cup chopped rhubarb
2 apples, peeled, cored, and sliced thin
2 tablespoons granulated sugar
2 tablespoons water

1. Preheat the oven to 325°F.

2. Lightly grease an 8-by-8-inch baking dish with butter; set aside.

3. In a small bowl, stir together the flour, sugar, and cinnamon until well combined.

4. Add the butter and rub the mixture between your fingers until it resembles coarse crumbs.

5. In a medium saucepan, mix together the rhubarb, apple, sugar, and water over medium heat and cook for about 20 minutes or until the rhubarb is soft.

6. Spoon the fruit mixture into the baking dish and evenly top with the crumble.

7. Bake the crumble for 20 to 30 minutes or until golden brown.

8. Serve hot.

PER SERVING Calories: 450; Fat: 23g; Carbohydrates: 60g; Phosphorus: 51mg; Potassium: 181mg; Sodium: 10mg; Protein: 4g

GINGERBREAD LOAF

Serves 16 / Prep time: 20 minutes / Cook time: 1 hour

Fragrant spices and a hint of sweetness make gingerbread a perfect choice for dessert any time of the year. The distinct flavor comes from the addition of fresh ginger. If you want to use ground ginger instead, add 1 tablespoon with the dry ingredients.

Unsalted butter, for greasing the baking dish
3 cups all-purpose flour
½ teaspoon Ener-G baking soda substitute
2 teaspoons ground cinnamon
1 teaspoon ground allspice
¾ cup granulated sugar
1¼ cups plain rice milk
1 large egg
¼ cup olive oil
2 tablespoons molasses
2 teaspoons grated fresh ginger
Powdered sugar, for dusting

1. Preheat the oven to 350°F.
2. Lightly grease a 9-by-13-inch baking dish with butter; set aside.
3. In a large bowl, sift together the flour, baking soda substitute, cinnamon, and allspice.
4. Stir the sugar into the flour mixture.
5. In medium bowl, whisk together the milk, egg, olive oil, molasses, and ginger until well blended.
6. Make a well in the center of the flour mixture and pour in the wet ingredients.
7. Mix until just combined, taking care not to overmix.
8. Pour the batter into the baking dish and bake for about 1 hour or until a wooden pick inserted in the middle comes out clean.
9. Serve warm with a dusting of powdered sugar.

PER SERVING   Calories: 232; Fat: 5g; Carbohydrates: 42g; Phosphorus: 54mg; Potassium: 104mg; Sodium: 18mg; Protein: 4g

ELEGANT LAVENDER COOKIES

Makes 24 cookies / Prep time: 10 minutes / Cook time: 15 minutes

There are more than 30 varieties of lavender, which can be grown in almost any area of the world with success. Lavender is not typically used in cooking, although it is edible and combines very well with many taste profiles. Lavender lends itself best to delicate desserts and baked items such as these elegant, buttery cookies.

5 dried organic lavender flowers, the entire top of the flower
½ cup granulated sugar
1 cup unsalted butter, at room temperature
2 cups all-purpose flour
1 cup rice flour

1. Strip the tiny lavender flowers off the main stem carefully and place the flowers and granulated sugar into a food processor or blender. Pulse until the mixture is finely chopped.

2. In a medium bowl, cream together the butter and lavender sugar until it is very fluffy.

3. Mix the flours into the creamed mixture until the mixture resembles fine crumbs.

4. Gather the dough together into a ball and then roll it into a long log.

5. Wrap the cookie dough in plastic and refrigerate it for about 1 hour or until firm.

6. Preheat the oven to 375°F.

7. Slice the chilled dough into ¼-inch rounds and refrigerate it for 1 hour or until firm.

8. Bake the cookies for 15 to 18 minutes or until they are a very pale, golden brown.

9. Let the cookies cool.

10. Store the cookies at room temperature in a sealed container for up to 1 week.

PER SERVING Calories: 153; Fat: 9g; Carbohydrates: 17g; Phosphorus: 18mg; Potassium: 17mg; Sodium: 0mg; Protein: 1g

CAROB ANGEL FOOD CAKE

Serves 16 / Prep time: 30 minutes / Cook time: 30 minutes

Angel food cake is a favorite of many people, especially in the summer months. Carob is a delicious substitution for cocoa powder that is lower in fat and higher in carbohydrates. This angel food cake would be fantastic paired with a cascade of fresh raspberries and topped with a dollop of whipped cream.

¾ cup all-purpose flour
¼ cup carob flour
1½ cups sugar, divided
12 large egg whites, at room temperature
1½ teaspoons cream of tartar
2 teaspoons vanilla

1. Preheat the oven to 375°F.
2. In a medium bowl, sift together the all-purpose flour, carob flour, and ¾ cup of the sugar; set aside.
3. Beat the egg whites and cream of tartar with a hand mixer for about 5 minutes or until soft peaks form.
4. Add the remaining ¾ cup sugar by the tablespoon to the egg whites until all the sugar is used up and stiff peaks form.
5. Fold in the flour mixture and vanilla.
6. Spoon the batter into an angel food cake pan.
7. Run a knife through the batter to remove any air pockets.
8. Bake the cake for about 30 minutes or until the top springs back when pressed lightly.
9. Invert the pan onto a wire rack to cool.
10. Run a knife around the rim of the cake pan and remove the cake from the pan.

PER SERVING Calories: 113; Fat: 0g; Carbohydrates: 25g; Phosphorus: 11mg; Potassium: 108mg; Sodium: 42mg; Protein: 3g

OLD-FASHIONED APPLE KUCHEN

Serves 16 / Prep time: 25 minutes / Cook time: 1 hour

Apfel kuchen *means "apple cake" in German. This version is a simple spiced cake studded with apples and served warm. Plums, peaches, pears, and berries can be substituted easily for the apples.*

Unsalted butter, for greasing the baking dish
1 cup unsalted butter, at room temperature
2 cups granulated sugar
2 eggs, beaten
2 teaspoons pure vanilla extract
2 cups all-purpose flour
1 teaspoon Ener-G baking soda substitute
2 teaspoons ground cinnamon
½ teaspoon ground nutmeg
Pinch ground allspice
2 large apples, peeled, cored, and diced (about 3 cups)

1. Preheat the oven to 350°F.

2. Grease a 9-by-13-inch glass baking dish; set aside.

3. Cream together the butter and sugar with a hand mixer until light and fluffy, for about 3 minutes.

4. Add the eggs and vanilla and beat until combined, scraping down the sides of the bowl, about 1 minute.

5. In a small bowl, stir together the flour, baking soda substitute, cinnamon, nutmeg, and allspice. ▶

6. Add the dry ingredients to the wet ingredients and stir to combine.

7. Stir in the apple and spoon the batter into the baking dish.

8. Bake for about 1 hour or until the cake is golden.

9. Cool the cake on a wire rack.

10. Serve warm or chilled.

PER SERVING Calories: 368; Fat: 16g; Carbohydrates: 53g; Phosphorus: 46mg; Potassium: 68mg; Sodium: 15mg; Protein: 3g

BUTTERY POUND CAKE

Serves 20 / Prep time: 20 minutes / Cook time: 1 hour, 15 minutes

Pound cake originated in Northern Europe. It got its name from the 1-pound measurements used for the ingredients—flour, butter, sugar and eggs. Cookbook measurements have since changed to cups, grams, and whole eggs, so the pound amounts are not as easy to notice. Over time, the original recipe also has evolved to include other ingredients such as sour cream, milk, baking soda, baking powder, and extracts for flavoring.

Unsalted butter, for greasing the baking pan
All-purpose flour, for dusting the baking pan
2 cups unsalted butter, at room temperature
3 cups granulated sugar
6 eggs, at room temperature
1 tablespoon pure vanilla extract
4 cups all-purpose flour
¾ cup unsweetened rice milk

1. Preheat the oven to 325°F.
2. Grease a 10-inch Bundt pan with butter and dust with flour; set aside.
3. In a large bowl, beat the butter and sugar with a hand mixer for about 4 minutes or until very fluffy and pale.
4. Add the eggs, one at a time, beating well after each addition and scraping down the sides of the bowl.
5. Beat in the vanilla.
6. Add the flour and rice milk, alternating in 3 additions, with the flour first and last.
7. Spoon the batter into the Bundt pan.
8. Bake for about 1 hour and 15 minutes or until the top of the cake is golden brown and the cake springs back when lightly pressed.
9. Cool the cake in the Bundt pan on a wire rack for 10 minutes.
10. Remove the cake from the pan to a wire rack and cool completely before serving.

PER SERVING Calories: 389; Fat: 20g; Carbohydrates: 50g; Phosphorus: 67mg; Potassium: 57mg; Sodium: 28mg; Protein: 5g

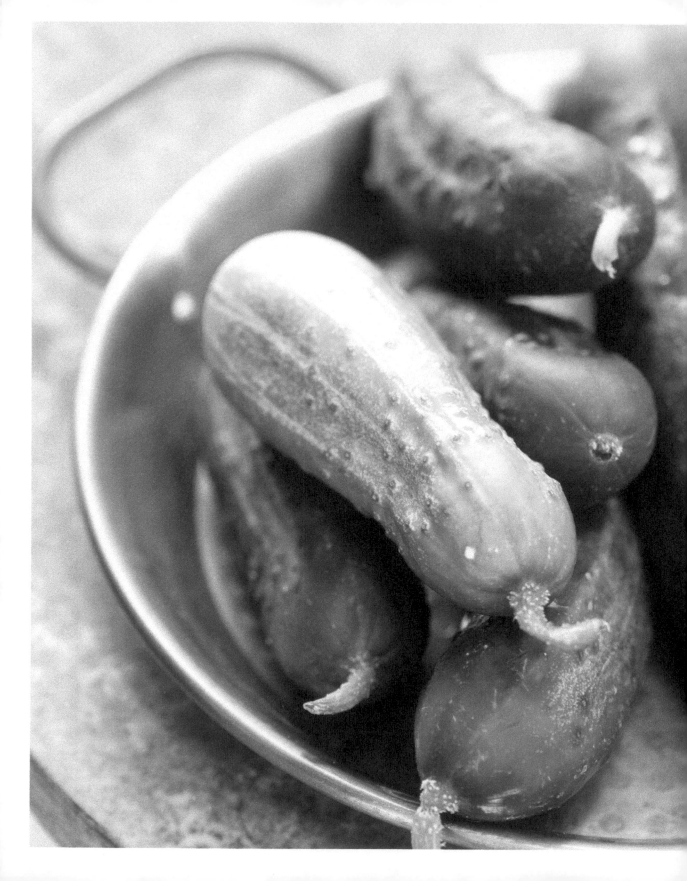

APPENDIX A
REFERENCES

American Diabetes Association. "Age, Race, Gender & Family History." February 12, 2014. Accessed June 15, 2015. http://www.diabetes.org/are-you-at-risk/lower-your-risk/nonmodifiables.html.

American Dietetic Association. "Pocket Resource for Nutrition Assessment: 2009 Edition." 2009. Accessed June 16, 2015. http://dpg-storage.s3.amazonaws.com/dhcc/resources/PocketResources/PRNA%202009.pdf.

American Kidney Fund. "Kidney Disease Statistics." Accessed June 14, 2015. http://www.kidneyfund.org/about-us/assets/pdfs/akf-kidneydiseasestatistics-2012.pdf.

American Kidney Fund. "Race/Ethnicity and Kidney Disease." Accessed June 15, 2015. http://www.kidneyfund.org/are-you-at-risk/risk-factors/race-kidney-disease.

Centers for Disease Control and Prevention. "National Chronic Kidney Disease Fact Sheet, 2014." 2014. Accessed June 16, 2015. http://www.cdc.gov/diabetes/pubs/pdf/kidney_factsheet.pdf.

Clinical Journal of the American Society of Nephrology. "Prevalence of Chronic Kidney Disease in US Adults with Undiagnosed Diabetes or Prediabetes." January 8, 2010. Accessed June 14, 2015. http://cjasn.asnjournals.org/content/5/4/673.

DaVita HealthCare Partners. "Phosphorus and Chronic Kidney Disease." Accessed June 18, 2015. http://www.davita.com/kidney-disease/diet-and-nutrition/diet-basics/phosphorus-and-chronic-kidney-disease/e/5306.

DaVita HealthCare Partners. "Potassium and Chronic Kidney Disease." Accessed June 18, 2015. http://www.davita.com/kidney-disease/diet-and-nutrition/diet%20basics/potassium-and-chronic-kidney-disease/e/5308.

Kidney & Urology Foundation of America. "High Blood Pressure and Kidney Disease." August 2005. Accessed June 16, 2015. http://www.kidneyurology.org/Library/Kidney_Health/High_Blood_Pressure_and_Kidney_Disease.php.

Krishnamurthy, V., G. Wei, B. Baird, M. Murtaugh, M. Chonchol, K. Raphael, T. Greene, S. Beddhu. "High Dietary Fiber Intake Is Associated with Decreased Inflammation and All-Cause Mortality In Patients with Chronic Kidney Disease." *Kidney International*, 81 (3: February 2012), 300–6. doi: 10.1038/ki.2011.355.

National Institute of Diabetes and Digestive and Kidney Diseases. "Kidney Disease of Diabetes." April 2, 2004. Accessed June 15, 2015. http://www.niddk.nih.gov/health-information/health-topics/kidney-disease/kidney-disease-of-diabetes/Pages/facts.aspx.

National Institutes of Health. "Kidney Disease: Early Detection and Treatment." *NIH Medline Plus* 3, no. 1 (winter 2008): 9–10. Accessed June 15, 2015. http://www.nlm.nih.gov/medlineplus/magazine/issues/winter08/articles/winter08pg9-10.html.

National Kidney Foundation. "About Chronic Kidney Disease." Accessed July 12, 2015. https://www.kidney.org/kidneydisease/aboutckd.

National Kidney Foundation. "Cholesterol and Chronic Kidney Disease." Accessed June 16, 2015. https://www.kidney.org/atoz/content/cholesterol.

National Kidney Foundation. "How Your Kidneys Work." Accessed June 15, 2015. https://www.kidney.org/kidneydisease/howkidneyswrk.

National Kidney Foundation. "KDOQI Clinical Practice Guidelines and Clinical Practice Recommendations for Diabetes and Chronic Kidney Disease." Accessed June 16, 2015. http://www2.kidney.org/professionals/KDOQI/guideline_diabetes/guide5.htm.

National Kidney Foundation. "Phosphorus and Your CKD Diet." Accessed June 16, 2015. https://www.kidney.org/atoz/content/phosphorus.

National Kidney Foundation. "Sodium and Your CKD Diet: How to Spice Up Your Cooking." Accessed June 17, 2015. https://www.kidney.org/atoz/content/sodiumckd.

National Kidney Foundation. "Vitamins and Minerals in Kidney Disease." Accessed June 17, 2015. https://www.kidney.org/atoz/content/vitamineral.

The Renal Association. "CKD Stages." Accessed June 16, 2015. http://www.renal.org/information-resources/the-uk-eckd-guide/ckd-stages#sthash.jWT6jJfH.dpbs.

Renal Health Network. "Are Your Kidneys Okay?" Accessed June 15, 2015. http://www.renalhealthnetwork.com/index.php?page=are-your-kidneys-okay.

US Department of Agriculture. "National Agriculture Library: Macronutrients." Accessed June 16, 2015. http://fnic.nal.usda.gov/food-composition/macronutrients.

US Department of Agriculture. "National Nutrient Database for Standard Reference Release 27." Accessed June 16, 2015. http://ndb.nal.usda.gov.

US National Library of Medicine. "Medline Plus: Chronic Kidney Disease." October 2, 2013. Accessed June 16, 2015. http://www.nlm.nih.gov/medlineplus/ency/article/000471.htm.

APPENDIX B
SHOPPING RESOURCES

I am lucky to live in a community where I have access to a variety of food-shopping sources, including farmers' markets and neighborhood and chain stores with organic and healthy offerings. Depending on where you are, this may not be the case. Here are some shopping resources that can help widen your food shopping possibilities.

Organic Local Produce

How do you know which food is organic? The United States Department of Agriculture (USDA) has strict production and labeling requirements when it comes to labeling organic foods. When something is labeled as 100 percent organic, it must meet the following requirements:

- All ingredients must be organic
- Any processing aids must be organic
- Product labels must state the name of the certifying agency on the food package

Many supermarkets now feature an organic section, but if yours does not, there are opportunities to find locally grown produce or have it delivered to you.

Farmers' markets and farm stands offer seasonal produce from organic and conventional farms. Produce is transported shorter distances and is generally grown using methods that minimize their impact on the earth. The fruits and vegetables you buy at the farmers' market are usually the freshest and tastiest available. You can find one closest to you using the Farmstand app (www.farmstandapp.com).

Community supported agriculture (CSA) programs deliver fresh produce several months out of the year. CSAs are often set up on a subscription plan; you pay a monthly fee for a weekly box of fresh produce from a local farmer.

Local Harvest (www.localharvest .org) is a good resource for finding farmers' markets and CSAs in your area. Their directory has more than 30,000 family farms and markets, along with restaurants and grocery stores that feature local food.

Natural food co-ops are another way to find local organic produce. Visit the Co-Op Directory Service (www .coopdirectory.org) to search for co-ops near you.

Door to Door Organics (www .doortodoororganics.com) makes online grocery shopping easy by quickly delivering fresh organic produce and local groceries to your home or office. Available in 13 states.

Organic Pastured Meats

Organic meats are made from animals that are fed food that doesn't contain any pesticides, chemicals, antibiotics, hormones, chemical fertilizers, or genetically modified organisms.

Eat Wild (www.eatwild.com) is an Internet database that helps you find local ranchers offering organic pastured meats and eggs. Some ranchers may sell the meat in bulk, whereas others sell at local farmers' markets, have stores on their property, or sell meats by the piece instead of by the whole animal or side.

US Wellness Meats (www.grasslandbeef .com) is an online retailer with a large selection of high-quality pastured animal products, including beef, pork, duck, buffalo, poultry, and wild-caught fish. The meats arrive in freezer containers over dry ice within two days.

RECIPE INDEX

INDEX

ACKNOWLEDGMENTS

I would like to express my gratitude to the many people who saw me through writing this book and to all those who provided support; talked through my ideas; read drafts; offered comments; and assisted with editing, proofreading, and design.

I would like to thank my family, especially my amazing siblings, who supported and encouraged me throughout the entire journey. I continue to be in awe of your support.

I would also like to thank Michelle Anderson, Peggy Perona, Robin Catalano, Jen Ross, Jean Stover, and Audrey Chapo for helping me in the process of selecting recipes and editing the drafts.

A special thanks goes to Meg Ilasco—without you, this book would have never found its way to me. Thank you so much for trusting me to write this book.

CPSIA information can be obtained
at www.ICGtesting.com
Printed in the USA
LVHW052039111021
700092LV00001B/2

9 781623 156619